BORN TO FLOURISH

Born to Flourish

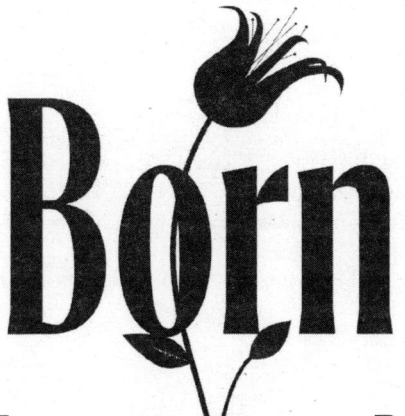

How New Science and Ancient Wisdom Reveal a Simple Path to Thriving

RICHARD J. DAVIDSON AND CORTLAND DAHL

SCRIBE

Melbourne | London | Minneapolis

Scribe Publications
18–20 Edward St, Brunswick, Victoria 3056, Australia
2 John St, Clerkenwell, London, WC1N 2ES, United Kingdom
3754 Pleasant Ave, Suite 223w, Minneapolis, Minnesota 55409, USA

Originally published by Avid Reader Press, an imprint of Simon & Schuster, LLC 2026
Published by Scribe 2026

Copyright © Richard J. Davidson and Cortland Dahl 2026

All rights reserved, including those for text and data mining, AI training, and similar technologies. Without limiting the rights under copyright reserved above, no part of this publication may be reproduced, stored in or introduced into a retrieval system, or transmitted, in any form or by any means (electronic, mechanical, photocopying, recording or otherwise) without the prior written permission of the publishers of this book.

The moral rights of the authors have been asserted.

Interior design by Ruth Lee-Mui

Printed and bound in the UK by CPI Group (UK) Ltd, Croydon CR0 4YY

Scribe is committed to the sustainable use of natural resources and the use of paper products made responsibly from those resources.

978 1 761381 33 1 (Australian edition)
978 1 917189 39 2 (UK edition)
978 1 761386 46 6 (ebook)

Catalogue records for this book are available from the National Library of Australia and the British Library.

scribepublications.com.au
scribepublications.co.uk
scribepublications.com

*To our teachers,
who offered us a glimpse of
what it means to truly flourish.*

Contents

Part 1: The Foundations of Flourishing   1

1. What Flourishing Is and Why It Matters   3
2. Rewiring Your Brain to Flourish   21
3. Flourishing in the Midst of Challenge   43
4. The Path to Flourishing   67

Part 2: The Four Skills of Flourishing   95

5. Awareness: The First Skill of Flourishing   97
6. Connection: The Second Skill of Flourishing   121
7. Insight: The Third Skill of Flourishing   147
8. Purpose: The Fourth Skill of Flourishing   175

Part 3: Flourishing Every Day   201

9. Making Flourishing a Habit   203
10. Change Your Mind, Change the World   219

Acknowledgments   231
Appendix: Additional Practices for Cultivating the Four Skills   235
Notes   261
Index   273

Part One

The Foundations of Flourishing

Chapter 1

What Flourishing Is and Why It Matters

> What lies behind us and what lies before us are tiny matters compared to what lies within us.
>
> —Ralph Waldo Emerson

Imagine you're walking along a wooded trail, your mind cluttered with the usual thoughts about work, relationships, and endless to-do lists. Suddenly, something catches your attention—perhaps a cluster of wildflowers swaying in the breeze or a shaft of sunlight breaking through the canopy. In that moment, everything shifts. Your mental chatter falls quiet. You feel deeply present, connected not just to the natural beauty around you but also to something larger than yourself. Time seems to pause, and you experience a profound sense of peace and purpose.

Most of us have experienced fleeting moments like these, moments when we break free from our constant doing and slip into a state of pure being. Maybe it happened during a heartfelt conversation where you felt truly seen and heard. Or perhaps while watching a sunset that took your breath away. In these rare moments, we catch a glimpse of what it means to truly flourish.

But here's the radical truth that decades of neuroscience research has revealed: these precious states don't have to be temporary. We can learn to flourish, even in the midst of our busy, modern lives. Even as depression rates soar, loneliness reaches epidemic levels, and attention spans dwindle in our hyperconnected world, we carry within us an innate capacity for profound well-being.

As longtime meditation practitioners, the two of us have discovered that flourishing isn't a matter of luck or circumstance—it's a skill that can be developed through practice, just like learning a language or playing a musical instrument. As scientists, we have discovered that you do not have to practice meditation to make this kind of lasting change. Through our work at the Center for Healthy Minds at the University of Wisconsin–Madison, we've identified four core dimensions, four core skills, that can be strengthened and enable us to thrive even in the face of life's greatest challenges.

Richie founded the Center for Healthy Minds in 2009 and the Dalai Lama visited Madison in 2010 to help inaugurate the Center. The mission of the Center is to cultivate well-being and relieve suffering through a scientific understanding of the mind. In 2014, Richie also founded Humin, a nonprofit company affiliated with the Center that has a mission to glean insights from the science to create tools to measure and disseminate well-being. Across these two organizations, there are about 100 people working to bring about a kinder, wiser, and more compassionate world. Both organizations working closely together is what fuels our secret sauce and allows us to uniquely contribute both fundamental science and practical tools that have impact.

Our research shows that just five minutes a day of practice can rewire your brain for greater resilience, focus, and well-being. In this book, we'll show you exactly how.

Humanity at a Tipping Point

The human species is experiencing a massive mental health crisis. Depression is now the leading cause of disease globally. Loneliness has been shown to be more dangerous to our health than smoking fifteen cigarettes a day. Suicide rates among different groups in some parts of the world are skyrocketing and cut across social class and income. Distractibility and impairments of concentration are also at an all-time high, and teens are spending more time on social media than they do sleeping. For the first time in US history, life expectancy is actually declining in parts of the population. Simply put, we are suffering.

How did we get here? Soon we will share the story of how we met, but for now, we arrived here through parallel complementary routes that included, for Richie, decades of scientific research and a sufficient taste of meditation to be convinced that it offers a powerful tool that can improve well-being; and for Cort, years in the Himalayas in Tibetan communities, learning Tibetan and Tibetan Buddhist practices, and thousands of hours on the meditation cushion. Together, as scientists and meditation practitioners, we've reached the simple yet powerful conclusion that flourishing needs to be nurtured, and from both the science and our personal experience, we have the strong conviction that it can be.

Richie is a neuroscientist and psychologist who began his career nearly fifty years ago with this question: Why is it that some people respond to life's slings and arrows with resilience, while others succumb to depression, stress-related disorders, and other forms of pathology? But it wasn't until 1992, when Richie first met the Dalai Lama, that he turned his attention fully to the study of the positive qualities in people, qualities such as compassion and wisdom.

Inspired by the Dalai Lama's advice and encouragement, in 2001,

Richie began a series of experiments in his lab with a group of very advanced meditation practitioners who had spent a significant portion of their adult lives in formal meditation retreats. One of the early visitors to his lab was Yongey Mingyur Rinpoche, then a very young Tibetan lama who had already logged more than 50,000 hours in formal meditation practice and had completed more than six years of retreat, meditating at least eight hours a day every day throughout those years. And it is largely because of Mingyur Rinpoche that we first met.

Cort's meditation journey began in the early 1990s when he was a college student struggling to cope with stress and anxiety. His passion for meditation led him on a journey around the world. He spent long periods in solitary retreat in the Himalayan foothills of Nepal, studied ancient meditation manuals with some of the most revered teachers of Tibetan Buddhism, and eventually cofounded Tergar, a global network of meditation centers spanning six continents, with Mingyur Rinpoche.

Despite our shared connection to Mingyur Rinpoche, we did not meet until 2010, when we attended a meeting with the Dalai Lama on "Altruism and Compassion in Economic Systems," hosted by the Mind & Life Institute in Zurich, Switzerland. Cort was attending with Mingyur Rinpoche, who had a deep interest in Western science and its connection to Buddhism. We heard about each other before we met, and we each sort of knew that we were destined to connect. When we first met, Cort was in the process of returning to the US after living in Asia for a decade. Our conversation rekindled his interest in science. Cort had studied psychology as an undergraduate, and he began to see how his background in both psychology and Buddhism could be combined in a doctoral study at the Center for Healthy Minds. By the end of the Zurich meeting, he'd decided to pursue his doctorate with Richie at the Center for Healthy Minds.

Our encounter in Zurich not only changed the course of Cort's life but also set the stage for a deep friendship and fruitful collaboration that continues to nourish us both and our joint commitment to work together on behalf of the well-being of others.

Beyond Mindfulness

Our very first conversations were filled with dreams of all the things we could explore together through the lens of scientific research. We were especially interested in broadening the scope of research beyond mindfulness, which was emerging as a hot topic in scientific circles at the time. The prevailing view was that mindfulness practice alone is the antidote to our stress and anxiety in an increasingly turbulent world. The basic idea is that by training the mind to stay in the present moment and develop greater calm and equanimity, we can weather life's storms with more resilience and feel better. Our intuition, however, was that while mindfulness skills are indeed critical for navigating the stress of the modern world, they would be even more impactful when paired with a broader range of contemplative principles.

This intuition has been borne out by our research. At the Center for Healthy Minds, we've found that mindfulness practice alone is not enough to reverse the trends we are seeing in people's mental health. As one of the premier centers for research into how meditation improves lives and the first to show that it actually changes the brain, the Center examines the effects of mindfulness and meditation—but our newest research has shown that something more is needed.

For the past four decades, we've investigated deeply the science of emotions and contemplative practice. We've studied attention, resilience, equanimity, kindness, compassion, gratitude, empathy, and wisdom, exploring how these qualities affect the mind, brain, and body.

Though we are scientists, we are also fathers, partners, and citizens who are not immune to the effects of the stress we are all experiencing. The suffering is all around us. As such, we developed a lofty goal. We wanted to see if we could help people achieve something concrete with this research, a path to thriving that would endure throughout their lives. We wanted to help people truly *flourish*.

In recent years, we have focused on two central questions: What skills do we need to flourish in the face of the increasing challenges of today's world? And is it possible to build our capacity to thrive when things are going well and to learn and grow and still be well when faced with enormous challenges? We've seen that flourishing comes about when:

1. we are fully present and aware,
2. we experience positive connections with the people in our lives and with the natural environment in which we reside,
3. we have insight into our thoughts and emotions, and
4. we feel that our lives have meaning and purpose.

And all this can still happen amid difficulty and stress.

Over the years, we've worked with thousands of people, from those struggling with depression and anxiety to stressed-out college students, from police officers to schoolteachers, and from newborn infants to aging adults. We've also studied the full range of psychopathology, from autism to depression, social anxiety, and PTSD, and we've explored the further reaches of human flourishing in very long-term meditation practitioners.

All along, we tracked the emotional lives of all these people, using the most cutting-edge research tools available, while giving them "behavioral tasks" (simple games) to study their behavior and well-being over time. We used magnetic resonance imaging (MRI), functional

MRI (fMRI), positron emission tomography (PET), and electroencephalography (EEG) to study their brains and found that meditation and other forms of mental training not only boost well-being but also alter the function and structure of the human brain, even how the brain responds to physical pain.

These measures helped us see that learning skills to cultivate flourishing makes us both feel better and behave more altruistically. Moreover, practices for flourishing help us stay more focused and can reduce unconscious biases. We used questionnaires and quizzes to see how skills for flourishing transform the way people think and feel about themselves. We also implemented biological measures that gave us insights into how training the mind can change how the physical body responds to stress—for example, decreasing the release of stress hormones during a challenging event.

These findings were surprising at times—and tremendously hopeful.

Our results showed that although the current trends around mental health are alarming, they *can* be reversed. Flourishing is possible amid a rapidly changing and busy world. What's more, we found that we all have the innate capacity to develop the skills and habits necessary to flourish. Learning to flourish is similar to learning language. But to actually do so, we need to be trained. Our big discovery is that flourishing consists of four skills. They can steer us away from depression and anxiety and toward fulfillment and connection. We can train ourselves to navigate life's ups and downs with far more resilience, calmness, and even a hopeful outlook. We can train our minds and rewire our brains to flourish.

The Four Skills of Flourishing

In this book, we give you practical steps for learning how to flourish in our everyday lives based on decades of research both in the lab and out in the world. We've examined brain scans and gene expression changes in the laboratory but also worked with people in real life who report profound shifts in well-being. We've worked with teachers, health care providers, police and firefighters, veterans, formerly incarcerated people, people suffering from mood and anxiety disorders, and many more. These skills are for all of us who are overwhelmed, stressed, or lonely in today's world or who simply sense they have untapped potential to lead a more fulfilling life. While our stress reactions are normal in a world of extraordinary challenge, it doesn't mean we can't train ourselves to thrive. Many of the people we have worked with reported feeling more depressed and anxious than ever before. Some said they no longer recognized themselves as the people they thought they were. Whether you live with chronic stress or mental health challenges are a new development for you, our book will illuminate the path from chronic stress, distraction, and anxiety to a life that feels balanced, rich, and rewarding.

We will share our groundbreaking scientific model—the Healthy Minds Framework—which highlights the *four core skills of human flourishing*. Each skill translates into practices that all of us can do in simple ways, every day, with enormous positive results.

Awareness: the skill of attending to the present moment and being with our own thoughts and emotions in a healthy way.

Connection: the skill of being present with others and our surroundings and the cultivation of qualities like appreciation and kindness that help us have healthy interactions and relationships.

Insight: the skill of building self-knowledge through self-inquiry, exploring how our thoughts, emotions, and sense of self shape our experience.

Purpose: the skill of feeling connected to the core values and guiding motivations that lend meaning to our lives and pursuits.

Our research on awareness, for instance, has shown that it plays a critical role in human flourishing by giving us the tools to manage our thoughts, emotions, and impulses in a healthy way—what scientists call "self-regulation." Our research on social connection has also led to striking results, including the finding that novice meditators can alter the functioning of their brains in ways that promote altruistic behavior. We found extraordinary examples of insight in advanced meditators, who could trigger and sustain high-amplitude gamma oscillations, a form of brain activity often associated with the experience of having an "aha" moment.

But by far, one of the most interesting aspects of our research is the role we learned purpose plays in flourishing. We would have thought that awareness, insight, and connection alone were enough to carry someone in times of great struggle—but, in fact, purpose plays a critical role. Purpose connects us to feeling needed and helps us keep our eye on creating a future we want to live in, which seems to lift us out of sadness and depression. While awareness, insight, and connection will keep us connected to our feelings and related capacities in the present moment, purpose pulls us into action. We've found that a healthy sense of purpose helps us recover more easily when we get emotionally reactive. People with more purpose are more emotionally resilient. If we translate this finding to a real-world setting, it means that on a day when you have more of a sense of meaning and purpose, you will more easily regain your emotional balance when you get upset or reactive.

Two Kinds of Learning

The four elements of flourishing we just introduced you to are called skills for a reason. For each of them, learning the skill requires not only conceptual learning about the skill but also practicing the skill to embody it. Consider kindness. You can read books about kindness and attend lectures about kindness. This is what's called didactic learning. It's how most of us were taught in school. But we all have a general intuition that while beneficial, just hearing about kindness is not sufficient to produce the feeling or act of kindness. For that we need *procedural learning*.

We've heard so many instances of people saying to us that they "know" they would benefit from meditating, but they still can't get themselves to do it. We see this pattern with other health-related behavioral changes we "know" would be good for us—better diets, more physical exercise, not smoking, etc. But we don't apply what we've learned to an effort to make the changes. Scientists call this the "declarative-procedural gap." Procedural learning is acquired through practice and it's procedural learning that enables us to establish a habit because it is governed by brain systems that are totally different from those that govern declarative learning.

Flourishing Is Easier Than You Think

Initially, we supposed that for the average person, cultivating the four skills would take hours of daily practice over the course of months and years. But when we studied the brains of both Buddhist monks who have meditated for tens of thousands of hours and those of everyday people just learning to meditate, we discovered our supposition was far from accurate. In fact, we don't even need to sit down to meditate for half an hour every day. According to our groundbreaking research, it only takes *a few minutes a day* of guided or unguided meditation, reflective writing, or short contemplation to rewire the brain to flourish.

To give just one of many examples, a study we did with hundreds of school employees at the height of the Covid-19 pandemic showed that doing the practices we teach in this book for just five minutes a day was enough to make substantial improvements in the participants' levels of stress and anxiety. Further, everyone reported an increase in positive thoughts and emotions, like feeling more aware and socially connected. What's more, these benefits started to show up after just one week of practice and were still present when we tested for them again three months after the program ended. And we now have very new data that show the benefits actually grow over time. In our six-month follow-ups, we've seen that the effects of the training are even more pronounced.

While our framework has been supportive for people during times of extreme stress, such as the Covid pandemic, it has also proven to help people with long-term mental health challenges. When we first met John, he was struggling with clinical levels of anxiety and depression and on the verge of quitting his job with the sales team at a big company. He enrolled in one of our studies at the Center for Healthy Minds and began to learn simple skills to work with his mind and emotions in a positive way. As early as the first week, he shared that he was feeling more hopeful and uplifted than he had in years. After a month, he started to feel more dramatic changes, and the data backed it up. His symptoms, including toxic levels of rumination and a lack of motivation to stay engaged at work, had decreased by nearly 30 percent. John reported higher levels of focus and mindfulness, more feelings of positive social connection, and a greater sense of meaning and purpose at work, all of which we were measuring weekly. The positive changes John experienced were still there three months later, and he shared that the training had transformed his life.

In other research using the most rigorous clinical research methods, we taught people who had never done any form of meditation training a simple compassion practice, which is important for both the awareness and connection aspects of flourishing and which we'll share in this book. This compassion practice asks participants to bring into their minds and hearts someone they know and to reflect on a difficulty that person is experiencing. The practitioner then cultivates a sincere wish that this person find happiness and be relieved of that difficulty. Participants are encouraged to begin this practice first by thinking of a loved one (a spouse, family member, even a pet), then they move on to someone they don't know very well, and, finally, to a challenging person in their lives. We tested participants before and after two weeks of this compassion training, with each person engaging in only seven hours total of practice.

What was most surprising is that we found evidence that the brain changed from pre- to post-training. Brain circuits critical for positive emotion became more activated. We also found that compared with a control group that did no compassion training, those trained in compassion acted more altruistically by giving generously to victims in an economic decision-making task. Altruism activates brain circuits and engages biological mechanisms of caring that contribute to our ability to flourish by helping us forge stronger connections with others. Together, these findings again confirmed that it doesn't take much training to measurably impact the brain circuits that underlie kindness and compassion.

The simplicity and accessibility of these practices are a seismic shift in our understanding of mental health and emotional well-being. If people adopt these habits and skills in the coming years, we can pave the way for huge reversals in declining mental health. We've seen that, like physical exercise, the four skills of flourishing are accessible to many, from kids in kindergarten to the elderly in nursing homes. Although we are taught to believe that people of a certain age are "too set in their ways" to change, this is simply not true. Research shows people can radically transform at any age. In one recent study, Anne Malaktaris and her colleagues at the University of California, San Diego, found that the compassion training we used in our studies produced substantial improvements in participants 66 years and older, showing significant gains in measures of well-being and decreases in measures of stress, anxiety, and feeling overwhelmed. Anyone can cultivate the skills of flourishing.

The four skills of flourishing can even influence how we respond to physical pain. In one of our studies, which we describe in detail later in the book, we found that cultivating awareness, connection, and insight changed the brain's pain network. Advanced meditators had much less activity in the pain network before and after a painful stimulus, while a group of nonmeditators experienced just the opposite. The takeaway is that we can train our minds to experience pain with less suffering. Imagine what the world would look like if we all learned the four skills of flourishing and applied them to the countless painful moments in our lives, both physical and otherwise.

All that is needed is a commitment to practice and a little bit of discipline for a few minutes each day. Brief daily rituals that help us calm our minds and live with more balance may one day be as common as brushing our teeth. Think about it. A few thousand years ago, humans were not brushing their teeth every day. This is something we learned to do. Now, virtually every person on the planet engages in this daily ritual. Consider what could happen if everyone cared for their minds daily the way we do for our bodies and physical hygiene. If each of us begins to incorporate these skills and habits into our daily lives, we imagine the alarming trends we are seeing will reverse, health will improve, and the effects will cascade to the flourishing of others in our communities and around the globe.

Flourishing Is Not Happiness

It is important to note that flourishing is not the same as being happy all the time. If you are helping a friend through a personal challenge, flourishing might look like empathy and being a present, caring listener. When you're at work, it might show up as mental focus, creativity, or staying connected to the deeper purpose of your job. And if you yourself are having a hard time, flourishing might look more like resilience, your capacity to adapt and adjust to an unexpected loss or a setback. Flourishing is the ability to see the forest from the trees and to remain buoyant, uplifted, and moving forward even during times of turbulence. In short, when we are flourishing, we bring the best of ourselves to whatever life throws our way.

The key insight from our pioneering research is the simple idea that flourishing is a skill. *Born to Flourish* will take you through a clear path that both explains the skills and the research behind them and that provides information on how you can nurture the skills in everyday life. When we take people through all four skills of the Healthy Minds Framework, the results are often life-changing.

For example, when we first started working with Jennifer, a forty-year-old public school teacher who was doing her best to help her class of unruly fifth-graders learn, she was on the edge of burnout. She loved teaching and her kids, but the daily grind of working in a large school system had created a feeling of chronic stress. Jennifer knew things were getting bad when she lost her ability to get a good night's sleep. She had always been a sound sleeper, but many nights she found herself lying in bed, staring at the ceiling. Her mind was caught in a swirl of thoughts, replaying stressful events from her day or imagining some unwelcome future scenario. Jennifer was exhausted yet couldn't fall asleep for hours, and when she did, she would wake up in the middle of the night with even more restless energy. Her fatigue started to spill over into her work and relationships. She couldn't stay focused in the classroom, and she was more irritable with her students. At home, the smallest chores started to feel like an overwhelming burden, and she lost the motivation to do things she normally enjoyed.

Jennifer had zero free time and was out of options, so based on a friend's recommendation, she downloaded our Healthy Minds Program app (produced by our nonprofit Humin), a step-by-step training in the four skills we cover in this book. Jennifer quickly discovered that the practices were much easier than she expected. She learned about "active meditations" she could do while folding the laundry or walking to the bus stop, and she learned she could practice while lying in bed, too. As she began integrating the skills into her life, things started to change.

In particular, the awareness practices helped her step back from the powerful current of her restless thoughts, emotions, and reactions. She learned how bringing awareness to the sensations of her body and breath as she lay in bed would bring a sense of peace and calm she'd never known before. She experimented with connection practices that taught her how to shift from frustration and apathy to empathy and appreciation. Insight meditation helped her explore her expectations and reactions with curiosity, and she started to feel much more in control of her emotions. She even learned some new skills to clarify her most cherished values and apply them when she was with her kids in the classroom, which helped her rediscover her passion for teaching. It was not an overnight process, but seeing that she could use the ups and downs of her daily routine to consciously strengthen awareness, connection, insight, and purpose transformed Jennifer's life at work and at home. Her story shows that it can take as little as five minutes a day to strengthen the four components of human flourishing.

The framework we founded and present in this book is the basis for the Healthy Minds Program app, which we developed together. The app has been selected as one of the top three meditation apps by *The New York Times/Wirecutter* for four years running and is being used in scientific research by some of the world's top scientists, including groups at MIT, NYU, the University of Wisconsin–Madison, the University of Arizona, and other premier universities. As of this writing it has been downloaded by more than one million people despite the fact that it was produced by a nonprofit organization that has spent nothing on advertising.

Unlike the app, however, this book isn't about practice alone. It brings stories, our research findings, and practices together in a single place to help you understand why we all struggle at times and how we can turn things around. Why do we handle a stressful work situation like a pro and then lose it sitting in traffic? Why do we feel a deep sense of purpose with some activities and not others? We've learned that variations in awareness, connection, insight, and purpose underlie all these fluctuations.

We are facing a crisis in our collective well-being today. Distractibility, addiction, loneliness, depression, suicide, and life expectancy are getting worse by the day. We need a reset! This is why the two of us consider ourselves "activist scientists." Seeing the growing scale of the mental health crisis and knowing what we know about simple skills that can help anyone flourish, we can no longer carry on with our research without acting. The world needs to know what the research is showing us: that simple practices to hone the four skills of flourishing can help us reverse the perilous course we are currently following as a society.

Born to Flourish aims to help each of us navigate the highs and lows of our individual lives and thereby thrive at work, at home, and everywhere in between. As we continue to face the stress and challenges around us, we ourselves can continue to change and increase our capacity to contribute good to the world.

Chapter 2

Rewiring Your Brain to Flourish

The privilege of a lifetime is to become who you truly are.

—Carl Jung

It was 7:30 a.m. on a crisp September morning when Cort pulled up to the drop-off line at Shorewood Elementary School with his eight-year-old son, CJ, sitting quietly in the back seat. As he watched CJ gather his oversized backpack and lunch box, Cort felt the familiar tightness in his chest—that mixture of love, worry, and determination that had become his constant companion over the past few months. Just a few months earlier, their lives had been completely upended. Now, here they were, starting an entirely new chapter in Madison, Wisconsin.

"Have a great day, hon," he said, trying to keep his voice steady. "Remember, Mrs. Johnson will take you to after-school care, and I'll pick you up at six after my classes." CJ nodded, gave him a quick hug, and disappeared into the stream of children flowing through the school's front doors. Cort sat there for a moment, watching him go, remembering how, just a year earlier, this whole routine would have played out back in Minneapolis, where Cort himself grew up and where all their family and friends were just a few minutes' drive away.

On this particular morning, the usual swirl of feelings Cort experienced when dropping off his son held an edge of something sharper—an awareness of just how much his life had changed in a matter of months. A difficult divorce had left him single-parenting CJ full-time, he'd just moved to a new city, and in a few days, he would be starting an intensive doctoral program. And then, just as he was adjusting to this new reality, came the news that his father had been diagnosed with cancer.

As he drove to campus for class, his phone buzzed. His father was calling with an update about his latest oncology appointment. The news wasn't good. It was stage 4 prostate cancer. The words still felt surreal, as if they belonged to someone else's story. Cort pulled into the parking lot on campus but couldn't bring himself to get out of the car just yet. The weight of everything—single parenting, the doctoral program's demanding schedule, his father's declining health, the geographic distance from their support system—felt as if it might crush him.

But sitting there in his car, he did what had become an essential part of his daily routine. He closed his eyes and allowed himself to feel the full weight of the moment. Some days, that meant tears. Other days, it meant feeling the anxiety course through his body like electricity. By bringing awareness to these feelings and feeling them fully, he'd discovered they would eventually pass on their own, leaving him better able to face whatever challenges lay ahead.

There were other supports Cort leaned on to get through this challenging time. He and CJ lived in family housing on campus, which was filled with kids and families who were also transplants, some much farther afield than Minneapolis. Seeing CJ play outside with new friends seemed to erase all of Cort's stress. But the most profound shifts happened in quiet moments—when CJ was missing his old room, his mom, or his friends. Instead of rushing to fix everything, Cort would simply be there with him. He learned that sometimes the most powerful thing he could do was just listen, acknowledging CJ's feelings without trying to make them go away. These moments, though difficult, deepened their bond in ways he hadn't anticipated.

Cort's relationship with his father had evolved, too. Their weekly calls, once focused on updates about treatment and test results, had transformed into deeper conversations about life, legacy, and what really matters. Despite the physical distance, Cort felt closer to his father than ever before. These conversations helped him see his own challenges through a wider lens, understanding that difficult periods often carry hidden opportunities for growth.

The daily juggle of responsibilities—making breakfast, reviewing scientific literature on his phone while waiting at soccer practice, working on papers after CJ went to bed—wasn't just about surviving. Each small action was part of a larger story about showing up for what matters most. When faced with competing demands, Cort found clarity by asking himself simple questions: *What kind of father do I want to be? What example do I want to set for CJ? What contribution do I hope to make through my research?*

Looking back on that period, the things that stood out weren't just the challenges but how they became opportunities for self-exploration and new insights and discoveries about life. The practices Cort learned over the years that helped him navigate this time weren't about eliminating difficulty—they were about developing a different relationship with it. Through daily moments of reflection, genuine human connection, and a deepening understanding of what truly matters, Cort discovered that it was possible to do more than just survive life's storms. It was possible to be transformed by them.

The tightness in Cort's chest that morning at CJ's school wasn't just anxiety. It was also the sensation of a heart expanding to hold both the pain and the possibility of their new life. Like any skill worth mastering, this ability to transform challenge into growth didn't come easily; it was the product of countless small choices, daily practices, and willing steps into uncertainty. Cort realized that flourishing is not a destination but a practice—one that asks only that we show up, stay present, and do our best to embrace life in all its complexity. The morning's familiar tightness wasn't just tension. It was the sensation of that practice at work, of a heart learning, through patient repetition, to turn life's hardest moments into opportunities for self-discovery.

We are all confronted by our anxieties, as Cort was during this critical period of his life. We get lost in distraction or depression, in fear or being overwhelmed, but we also carry the seeds to flourish, even though many of us are simply not aware we have these capabilities. Sometimes, when we encounter a person who is especially compassionate or wise, they help us recognize these qualities in ourselves. Maybe you feel a heart connection or like you've known them forever even though you just met. We often describe these encounters as heartwarming.

Feelings of connection are one surefire way to flourish, but there are many others. Think about a time when you felt attentive, focused, and at ease in the present moment. Perhaps you were in nature and experienced awe in response to natural beauty. What did that moment feel like to you? What was the trigger that allowed you to access this deep sense of flourishing?

The moments of serenity Cort experienced after his son CJ went to sleep or when he was by himself in his car in the parking lot were glimpses into the experience of deep flourishing. Cort could not help but wonder: *What if this state could become more frequent and enduring? Is it possible for us to cultivate a state of flourishing in any situation? Could we rewire ourselves to strengthen these qualities, the way we strengthen the heart and other muscles with physical exercise? And like learning to play a musical instrument, could we practice and get better at flourishing?*

What does it mean to flourish? As we said in the first chapter, flourishing has four essential components: Awareness, Connection, Insight, and Purpose. We are flourishing when we are fully present with ourselves and our surroundings, connected to those around us and to our context, understand how our beliefs and expectations of ourselves shape our experience of the world, and have a sense of purpose that goes beyond ourselves.

Soon after we first met, we recognized we had something big in common: a shared conviction that humans are born to flourish and that everyone has the capacity to change.

The Pliable Brain and Body

Our brains and bodies are wired for change. Neuroplasticity refers to our brain's capacity to form new neural pathways, even entire networks, when we learn something. For example, if you learn a visual-motor skill like juggling, which requires precise hand-eye coordination, the pathways between the visual and movement centers in your brain will be measurably strengthened. The next time you try to juggle will be easier because you created these new pathways.

Epigenetics studies the way a modification to a gene changes the gene's expression. For example, in our laboratory, we've demonstrated that just one day of intensive meditation practice among long-term meditation practitioners results in an epigenetic change that decreases the body's inflammatory molecules. This decrease in inflammation, a common factor in many chronic illnesses, shows that the habit of meditation changes how a person's genes are expressed.

Even though we are wired for change, it doesn't mean we always change for the better. Throughout our lives, we can change in ways that make us angrier, more fearful, more distracted, more detached and alone, and unhappier—the opposite of flourishing. If we build a habit of doomscrolling our social media feeds every day, our brains will wire toward that habit. If we build a habit of going into a rage every time we sit in traffic, we will wire that habit. But here's the good news: the very same aspects of our biology that can be hijacked to produce suffering can be harnessed for our good and help us flourish.

Sculpting the Brain

Have you ever marveled at the changes that babies show over the first three years of development? How do we go from fragile, preverbal infants who sleep most of the time to curious, hyperverbal toddlers? What about watching with breathtaking wonder how an Olympic figure skater accomplishes the near-impossible jumps that mesmerize global audiences? Or listening with reverence to a virtuoso musical performance? In each of these cases, the skills these infants, athletes, and musicians display are a product of their neuroplasticity. In acquiring these skills, the brain is sculpted by experience and training. These neuroplastic changes establish a new baseline, so that the next time a toddler, athlete, or musician performs, the skilled behavior will unfold ever more seamlessly.

Changes in our brains can occur wittingly or unwittingly. Most of the time, neuroplastic changes occur unwittingly. Our brains are constantly being shaped by the forces around us, and we are usually oblivious to these changes. A common yet unfortunate example is the prevalent fear-based advertising we see during a US election season. Doctored images of "immigrants" committing crimes, for example, likely hijack the brain's fear circuit and lower its threshold for activation. We're not aware that our brains are being sculpted by these experiences, but evidence shows that they are. In this case, the threshold for activating our amygdala—an important emotional center in the brain—might be lowered so that innocuous events might trigger it and be experienced as threats.

But we can also alter our brains wittingly by training our minds, much the same way training the body through physical exercise leads to changes in the immune system and other aspects of our physical health. For example, your brain will change by engaging in a simple awareness practice like noticing your breath and returning your attention to it every time you get distracted. The more you do this, the more you will strengthen this new neural connection, which reinforces the habit. Before you know it, you will be less distracted and use your breath to help yourself focus without even thinking about it. Another simple way to train your mind is with the practice of appreciation. Have you ever paused for a few moments to appreciate nature? Or the positive qualities of another person? If you do this consciously and repeatedly, it will induce a neuroplastic change that results in appreciation arising more spontaneously in the future.

We need to be intentional about how we engage with the world and pick up the skills we need to improve our well-being. Otherwise, our neuroplastic brains will be hijacked by the forces around us, and we'll find ourselves with all sorts of habits that increase suffering. It isn't easy. To paraphrase a bumper sticker frequently spotted in the US, "Stuff happens." Adversity is all around us; it's a part of life. We cannot buffer ourselves from it completely. By training our minds, however, we can change our relationship to adversity and transform the difficult periods of life into opportunities for learning and growth.

When a stressful challenge occurs, it triggers a cascade of changes in the brain and body. Imagine having an argument with your partner, your child, or a friend early in the morning. The sight and sounds of the interaction will be registered by the visual and auditory cortices—the parts of your brain that process information from your eyes and ears. Each of these sensory-specific brain regions has a pathway of connecting neurons to the amygdala—that major processing center for our emotions that is triggered when something important happens. If it's something positive, it would be good to keep it going and savor whatever is happening. But when it's a stressful event, other parts of the brain become engaged to help formulate a plan to decrease the stress. The plan might be to try to escape the situation, or it might be to reinterpret the situation so that it becomes less stressful.

The early-morning argument will also affect your body. Our brains are neuroplastic, and you might say that our bodies are plastic, too. That probably sounds really strange, but it simply means that our bodies, like our brains, are constantly changing and adapting to our current circumstances. When you're in an argument, your body becomes stressed as it receives signals from the brain. One of the key structures transmitting information from the brain to the body is the insula, which lies near the front of the brain, behind your forehead. The insula is the only part of the brain that contains what we call a "viscerotopic map." In other words, many of our major bodily organs, including the heart, lungs, and sex organs, are mapped onto geographic regions of the insula. During and after the argument with your loved one, when the insula is activated, your breathing may become more rapid, and your heart may beat more quickly and strongly so that you feel heart palpitations. This is how your insula is literally talking to your heart and lungs.

Your heart and lungs, in turn, talk to your brain. The pathways between the insula and the visceral organs of the body are not one-way. William James, America's first great psychologist, famously proposed that an emotion is the perception of a bodily change. So, in our example of the morning argument, when your brain perceives the acceleration of your breathing and heart rate, you might experience anxiety or fear. This pattern in the body coordinates with a pattern in the brain that might activate the salience network, which in turn ramps up these bodily changes. The salience network incorporates brain regions that function to label activities and events that are significant, like emotional events that are personally meaningful so that our emotions leave memory traces in our bodies and brains.

When we cultivate the qualities of flourishing, we're not only changing our minds but also altering our brains, which, in turn, will impact our bodies. Just as the body can tense in response to stress and form body memories around struggle, the reverse is also true. When the body is in a calm state and breathing is slow, it will bathe the brain in soothing neural impulses and help quiet the structures involved in the fight-flight-freeze response, and that state of calm in the brain will inform the body.

The Machinery of Plasticity

But let's back up because it will be helpful to look more deeply at how plasticity works so you can appreciate the miraculous machinery of what it means to be human. Our nervous system enables us to sense, feel, breathe, think, move, create, and imagine.

The nervous system's basic building block is the nerve cell, or neuron. A neuron is designed to send and receive messages between two or more parts of the brain or between the brain and the body. Including the brain, spinal cord, and the rest of the body, we have approximately 135 billion neurons at any given time. Each of the five senses has specialized neurons: neurons responsible for vision are in our eyes, those responsible for smell are in our nose, and so on. And we have motor neurons specialized to produce action.

We also have interneurons, nerve cells dedicated to forming connections. These little cells are the fundamental building block of neuroplasticity. Unlike simpler organisms, humans have brains in which most nerve cells are these interneurons. In other words, we can form connections between our senses, movements, ideas, thoughts, and feelings far more than any other living organism can. Another way of saying this is that we have a greater ability to learn new skills than other living creatures.

Interneurons grow and change in response to experience and training. In a famous study published twenty-five years before the widespread use of GPS and Google Maps, a group of neuroscientists at University College in London looked at the brain anatomy of London taxi drivers. They wanted to see if learning to navigate the complex streets of London would induce measurable changes in the parts of the brain essential for memory and spatial navigation. For those who've been to the city of London, you know that navigating its curved and narrow streets is like learning a second language. Becoming a London taxi driver usually requires two full years of training to pass the mandatory police exam, which includes navigation. Using a structural MRI scan, the study compared the brain anatomy of experienced London taxi drivers with inexperienced drivers of the same age and gender. Researchers were particularly interested in the hippocampus, an elongated structure on each side of the brain, buried within the temporal lobe, the part of the brain just above the ears. They found that the size of the posterior portion of the hippocampus was significantly larger in the experienced taxi drivers compared with the inexperienced drivers, and the longer a driver had been driving, the larger this area of the hippocampus.

It turns out that the hippocampus is one of the essential brain regions for flourishing. Researchers have shown that simple awareness-based meditation practices increase the volume, the literal size, of the hippocampus. Given its role in memory, this brain region is important in helping us remember to bring a flourishing mindset to our everyday interactions.

The taxi driver study was one of the first of a small cottage industry of research suggesting that when we use a specific part of the brain extensively to develop a particular expertise, that part of the brain gets larger. The connections between that area and other areas of the brain also increase.

Learning the skills of flourishing similarly induces changes in the brain, as the research with simple awareness meditation has demonstrated. In a study at the Center for Healthy Minds, Tammi Kral, a graduate student at the time, examined possible changes in the neuronal connections between different brain regions using training in a simple awareness practice (stay tuned for chapter 5). In particular, she wanted to know if an eight-week awareness training would alter the actual neuronal connections between the network in the brain responsible for rumination and mind-wandering (called the default mode) and the network responsible for directing attention and self-regulation (known as the central executive network).

The study participants were randomly assigned to either eight weeks of awareness meditation training or one of two different control groups. One control group was called the Health Enhancement Program, a training we invented to control for the group experience, which promised some benefit and an enthusiastic instructor. The awareness training group and the Health Enhancement Program group were perfectly matched on each of the dimensions. The other control group was a "wait-list" control, which was told they could take either the awareness training or the Health Enhancement training after six months.

In the group practicing meditation, we found increased connectivity between the two important networks in the brain. The conclusion here is that training in simple mindful awareness (which is part of the awareness pillar we teach later in the book) does help us direct our attention and regulate mind-wandering. The fact that a modest dose of awareness meditation training—in this case approximately twenty-four hours spread across eight weeks—produces measurable structural brain changes in the connections between these two important networks underscores that we can all change our brains, and therefore our lives, with just a bit of mental training.

It wasn't long ago that scientists held a very different view. When Richie was a graduate student, he was taught that the brain could not generate new cells, unlike other parts of the body. We all know that if we injure our skin, new cells will grow back to replace the damaged skin. Until 2000, everyone believed humans are born with all the neurons we'll have in our lifetime. People thought that infants are born with more neurons than they need and that their cells are "sculpted" as they develop. In other words, cells that are not required for a specific task die off. But it turns out that thinking was wrong. Our brains are generating new cells all the time.

We now know that adult humans grow an average of 1,000 new neurons daily, and we also know that unhealthy states of mind, like stress and depression, impair our ability to grow new neurons. The growth of new neurons is important for flourishing. By engaging in some key healthy habits of mind (which we'll share in subsequent chapters), we can harness the potential for change in our brains and bodies in ways that support enduring flourishing. Once you begin to see that you carry within you the potential to change for the better and that these transformations of mind will literally change your brain and improve its health, a new sense of hope emerges for what may be possible in the future.

Our Genes Have Volume Controls

Like neuroplasticity, epigenetics is a relatively new but very powerful way of understanding our potential for change. We all have genes that predispose us to one or another trait, but the extent to which a gene is expressed (that is, turned up or down like a volume control) determines the extent to which its trait is expressed. For example, if you have a gene from your father that predisposes you to anxiety, but your genetically unrelated caregiver is very laid-back and relaxed, you could experience an epigenetic change that "turns down the volume" of the anxiety-related gene you inherited from your father. The change can down-regulate the anxiety-related gene so that it produces less of the stress hormone cortisol, for example.

The extent to which any given gene is expressed is influenced by a host of factors, including internal stressors, such as our emotions, and environmental stressors. Just because we carry a gene that might predispose us to a disease—the APOE4 gene, which is connected to Alzheimer's disease, for example—it doesn't mean that gene will be turned up or activated. We can live with the gene for a disease and never get that illness. Take, for example, two people with identical genetic risk for Alzheimer's. Research shows that if a person is very active intellectually—reading, writing, engaging in discussions about theater, art, or politics—that person will, all other things being equal, have a less severe presentation of the illness.

Think of each of your genes as having a volume control that goes from low to high. This volume control determines how much protein a gene will produce, and whether or not the protein is manufactured will determine the expression of that gene. For example, if a gene that produces a protein to increase inflammation is not activated, it will keep inflammation at low levels.

Many factors can influence the volume control on our genes, from our emotions to our life circumstances. For example, research shows that environmental factors like trauma have a huge impact on the volume control of our genes. What is even more amazing is that such effects can be passed down at least a couple of generations. Rachel

Yehuda, a neuroscientist at Mount Sinai School of Medicine in New York City, has been studying the neuroscience of stress for decades. In 2016, she and her colleagues published a groundbreaking article about the epigenetics of stress in a group of 32 Holocaust survivors and 22 of their adult children. Their research included a demographically matched control group of parents and children not exposed to the Holocaust. Among both the Holocaust survivors and their children, researchers found an alteration in the epigenetic status of a gene that plays a critical role in regulating the neurochemicals involved in our response to the stress hormone cortisol. No such alteration was found in the control group. In other words, the participants who had experienced the unimaginable traumas of the Holocaust and their children both carried a biological alteration that predisposed them to even more dysregulation in their hormonal responses to stress.

Gene expression is also affected by our circadian rhythms. When we transition from waking to sleep and then back again, a host of genes are up- and down-regulated. Some of these genes regulate the sleep-wake cycle itself. Other genes triggered in the sleep-wake transition are involved in inflammation, which suggests that sleep (particularly deep sleep) can have an anti-inflammatory effect. Interestingly, these patterns are disrupted in patients with certain major psychiatric disorders such as schizophrenia.

The simple fact that our genes are up- and down-regulated during sleeping and waking is a fascinating little detour—which *is* related to flourishing. When we are stressed, we lose sleep, and that loss of sleep can activate gene expressions that further our inflammation and stress.

Through our work at the Center for Healthy Minds, we realized that if trauma and our circadian rhythms can exert epigenetic effects and be passed down from generation to generation, it was highly likely that mental training to promote flourishing could alter our epigenetics in a positive direction—which leads us to believe that the qualities of flourishing can also be transmitted intergenerationally. An amazing possibility and an inspiration to all current and future parents!

One of the key collaborators in our epigenetics and flourishing research is an extraordinary woman named Perla Kaliman. We call Perla "the wandering yogi scientist." Originally from Argentina, where she received a doctorate in biochemistry, and a professor and researcher at the University of Barcelona in Spain, Perla travels the world harnessing opportunities to engage in collaborative work and relieve suffering. Along with Perla, Antoine Lutz, a French neuroscientist; Melissa Rosenkranz, one of the Center's core faculty members; and Richie designed a novel study with 19 long-term meditation practitioners, including Cort before he moved to the Center to pursue his doctorate. The meditation practitioners came to our lab for a full day of intensive meditation practice that included both sitting and walking practice. They were compared with 21 nonmeditating control participants who also came to the lab for a "day of leisure" that included quiet activities such as reading, watching videos, and walking. The duration of practice or leisure for both groups was 8 hours.

At the beginning and end of the day (8 a.m. and 4 p.m.), blood samples were obtained, and white blood cells were extracted for epigenetic analysis. DNA methylation is a process that dynamically influences gene expression. We searched for genes that were differentially methylated between pre- and post-day intervention in the meditators versus the controls. We found 61 genes that met rigorous criteria for differential methylation between the meditators and controls, and it turned out that most of these genes were in pathways critical for the regulation of inflammation. The meditators were showing a downregulation of genes implicated in inflammation. This is remarkable since it occurred over the span of only 8 hours.

Many chronic illnesses include inflammation as a key component of the illness, ranging from asthma to inflammatory bowel disease to many forms of cardiovascular disease. Even Alzheimer's and other forms of dementia involve inflammation—in this case, in the brain. These facts invite the exciting possibility that nurturing human flourishing might not only benefit psychological well-being but also physical health, particularly in people who suffer from inflammatory illnesses.

Born to Flourish

In a nutshell, neuroplasticity and epigenetics can work for or against us in our ability to flourish. But there is a third internal mechanism that always works in our favor: what we call innate goodness. Innate goodness helps us make choices that make a positive impact on our minds and epigenetics.

Cort saw this innate propensity for goodness firsthand when he lived with his family in Nepal. Cort's son, CJ, was born in Kathmandu and spent his early years playing in the shadow of the towering Boudhanath Stupa, an ancient Buddhist monument on the outskirts of the Kathmandu Valley. The Tibetan refugee community had settled in this area decades earlier. In what would eventually become their daily ritual, Cort took CJ out each morning and evening for the traditional circumambulation of the massive Buddhist monument, a centuries-old Tibetan practice. Together, they joined throngs of Tibetan monks and nuns, local Nepalis, and Tibetan refugees as they slowly walked in a clockwise circle around the stupa.

The bustling pathway was often lined with beggars—elderly men and women with weathered faces, children with outstretched hands, and others, often draped in tattered clothing. To many, they might have seemed an intimidating or uncomfortable presence, but to CJ, they were simply people in need. While some young children might shy away from unfamiliar faces and cling fearfully to their parents, CJ displayed a remarkable instinct that transcended his limited life experience. Barely able to walk and not yet speaking, he would purposefully approach these strangers seeking alms, and, without prompting, he would reach into Cort's pockets searching for anything that could be shared—coins, small items, or bits of food. If he found nothing to give, he would point insistently toward nearby shops, his gesture clearly communicating a desire to acquire something not for himself but to share with others.

What made CJ's behavior so striking was the pure, unlearned quality of his compassionate impulses. In a stage of life traditionally marked by the refrain "mine!" and requests for treats and toys, CJ's natural inclination was toward giving rather than receiving. His spontaneous generosity emerged before any formal teaching about sharing or kindness, suggesting something more fundamental at work.

CJ's instinctive compassion in the streets of Kathmandu points to a profound truth about human nature that science is only beginning to fully understand. As we'll see, research now reveals that this innate orientation toward goodness isn't a heartwarming anomaly—it's a fundamental aspect of human development that manifests long before cultural conditioning or social learning can explain it. We're discovering that while our brains and genes can be influenced in many directions, there exists within us a natural compass that points toward kindness, connection, and flourishing.

As Cort observed in his son, we all come into the world with a preference for goodness. We are drawn to kindness, openness, and relaxation, to a smile rather than a grimace. We yearn to live a life of joy and purpose and to connect with both ourselves and others. This preference, this yearning, has the power to direct us.

The notion of basic goodness may sound unscientific, but this principle is rooted in rigorous and methodical research. One body of work has shown that infants are oriented toward kindness even before they've had the opportunity to learn about social preferences. In 2007, a group of psychologists at Yale conducted an experiment in which six-month-old infants sat on their mother's lap in front of a contraption designed for this experiment, a wooden incline on which a stick figure with eyes was placed. The children watched as the figure appeared to climb but twice got stuck two-thirds of the way up. In a third scenario, another figure came to help the first figure and push it up the hill. In a fourth, a different-colored figure appeared to push it down the hill. The experimenters measured how long infants gazed at each of these figures as a measure of their preference.

Among the six-month-old infants, 100 percent preferred the helper. In some ways, this result might seem unremarkable, but is remarkable—the infants were so young they had not yet been taught social norms of any kind. The finding indicates that even as infants we carry an overwhelming and seemingly universal preference for goodness. We prefer warmhearted, kind, and altruistic interactions to selfish and aggressive ones. Tapping into this innate drive will help us cultivate the skills to flourish.

Infants also show an innate disposition to help relieve others' distress. In other words, we are all born with what we might call innate compassion. In a research study we conducted in our lab in collaboration with developmental psychologist Hill Goldsmith in the late 1990s, we tested 368 toddlers at 32 months of age. The study was primarily focused on behavioral inhibition, or shyness, in children.

In one part of our research, a staff member held an old-style clipboard and, at some point, feigned getting her finger stuck in the clipboard clip, grimacing and verbalizing an "ouch!" The toddlers were videotaped during this interaction to ascertain their responses. Viewing the short video clips of all 368 toddlers and observing the behavioral range in their response to this situation was remarkable. The vast majority of toddlers attempted to relieve the experimenter's distress. Some asked the experimenter if she was okay, others asked if she needed a bandage, and still others kissed the experimenter's finger. More than two-thirds of the toddlers this age displayed some form of helping behavior.

Kiley Hamlin, a psychologist at the University of British Columbia, who is an early pioneer in studies on innate goodness, points to three characteristics of infants that convincingly reveal our innate capacity to flourish:

Infants show a moral goodness in their propensity to help others in distress.

Infants have the capacity for moral understanding and evaluation. They understand social interactions, evaluate them, and show a clear preference for altruistic and warmhearted social interactions.

Infants exhibit a preference for moral retribution. If an actor is selfish and mean to others, they want to see such "bad guys" get punished. This preference has been demonstrated in infants as young as five months.

The combination of these three characteristics provides the young infant with an innate moral compass and a core foundation for flourishing throughout their lives. It also suggests that when we teach simple practices to cultivate qualities such as compassion, which enhances our connection with others, we are not generating these qualities de novo but rather are familiarizing ourselves with the basic nature of our minds and strengthening these innate qualities.

The fact that goodness is innate is hugely important. It tells us that the qualities of kindness we seek to cultivate are qualities we already have. They simply need to be recognized and strengthened. This was a very important insight for us and directly contributed to the formulation we present in this book.

The Importance of Intention

Each of us is born with the seeds of flourishing. For these seeds to grow, however, we need to nurture them by taking advantage of the building blocks that can help change our brain structure. In the following chapters, we will take you through the four key components essential to nurture these seeds into full bloom. As they grow, you will find yourself flourishing, even during times of stress. This is tremendously hopeful news. The study of the brain and our innate ability to change for the better is essentially a science of hope. We just need to tap into our brain's capacity to rewire, our capacity to influence our genes, and the orientation toward goodness that has been with us since the beginning.

Even as our brains and the expression of our genes are always changing in response to our shifting circumstances, we can nurture our innate capacities to flourish and thrive with simple practices. It really just comes down to making a choice, and an intentional mindset helps. If we can be intentional about our brains and bodies as we direct our minds toward habits and behaviors, we can support our flourishing. We do not have to default to the habits dictated by our surroundings.

PRACTICE

Morning Moments of Appreciation

Here's a simple exercise to try for a week: every morning, while brushing your teeth, bring a loved one into your mind and heart. It could be a spouse, a child, another family member, or a dear friend. As you hold this person in your mind and heart, recall something specific and positive about them. It could even be something small, like how this person always says thank you when receiving something. Whether large or small, simply focus on a positive attribute.

At the end of the week, check in with yourself and notice how this exercise has altered your state of mind. You will likely discover two things. First, it doesn't take much to orient the mind toward the positive, and that positive feeling may carry over into your day. You might even find that this small change impacts your ability to flourish on any given day. Second, you will likely notice that even this simple and short practice is filled with distraction. Maybe your dog barked or a child called out, and you started thinking about a million other things. Maybe your phone dinged, and you remembered that call you forgot to return. In today's world, we are bombarded with distractions.

Distraction is one of the major obstacles to flourishing. It deserves our attention and will be a focus for exploration in the next chapter. What are we up against as we take on the commitment to nurture flourishing? Understanding the obstacles and forces that promote suffering is key to the solution.

Chapter 3

Flourishing in the Midst of Challenge

Strength does not come from physical capacity, it comes from an indomitable will.

—Mahatma Gandhi

Erik Olin Wright was a well-known professor of sociology at the University of Wisconsin–Madison where we work, a former president of the American Sociological Association, and a dear friend of Richie's. In 2019, he passed away at the age of seventy-one from an advanced form of leukemia.

The year before his passing, Erik lived much of the time at Froedtert Hospital, just outside Milwaukee, where he received bone marrow transplants and other advanced treatments for the aggressive cancer eating away at his body. The treatment was brutal. When they removed his cancer-ridden bone marrow and replaced it with transplanted marrow, Erik needed to be in an isolated, germ-free room. When he received radiation, he experienced brain fog and incredible fatigue, a very different experience for someone with the energy of a spark plug. Erik was always vivacious, enthusiastic, and passionate about his work and family.

Although the combination of the treatment and the effects of the illness were devastating, Erik managed to flourish. It would be easy to think that he and others like him somehow rise above their gruesome circumstances because of some genetic predisposition. While Erik might have had some resilience genes that helped him, and though he'd had a happy childhood, it was clear to Richie that the active ingredient in his flourishing was that he trained himself through writing, meditation, and making a very intentional commitment to the many friendships he maintained with former students and colleagues from around the world.

While he was ill, Erik kept a journal that he originally intended would inform his friends and family about the medical events he was experiencing as they occurred. He distributed this personal journal to a group of at least fifty close friends. The journal quickly expanded beyond the medical details to include his thoughts, emotions, and perspective on his mortality.

Earlier in Erik's life, he had decided to take a mindfulness meditation course and begin a daily meditation practice. He considered it so valuable that he went on to start all the classes he taught with a short meditation practice, including his wildly popular course Contemporary American Society, which had an enrollment of at least four hundred students every year. The skills Erik learned from his meditation practice came in handy when the challenges of his leukemia became acute.

Richie had the privilege of being with Erik the day before he passed in his hospital room in Milwaukee. Erik talked about love as the essential ingredient in human relationships. Although he had endured a brutal six-month stay in the hospital, on this day, the day before his passing, Erik was flourishing. He was keenly aware of what was happening to his body, his circumstances, and his very finite timeline, yet he radiated love for his family, friends, and the strangers in the hospital who quickly became his friends. His purpose in life could not be stronger. Erik was intensely curious and wise and flourished even as he was dying. We might even say he was in an optimal state of flourishing because he was dying.

Why Are We So Anxious, Overwhelmed, and Depressed?

This story of Erik's final days points to an important truth about the human experience: there are moments in life when intense challenges and unexpected setbacks bring out our very best. These are times when we rise above our circumstances. We may even surprise ourselves by the degree of our courage and resilience. Life challenges may not be pleasant, but they can be deeply transformative. They can even lead to major insights about life or a recalibration of our priorities.

This may sound like good news, but unfortunately, the reverse is also true. The difficult moments of life can completely knock us off balance, and when difficulties never seem to end, they can leave us feeling depleted and overwhelmed. Indeed, many of us are living in a state of chronic stress these days. On top of all the massive challenges we face as a species, we are all doing our best to cope with work stress, health issues, relationship difficulties, and the daily grind of a to-do list that never seems to end.

We are living through a unique period in human history in which many of the factors that support our ability to flourish are in short supply, while many of those that undermine it surround us on all sides. It may be depressing, but seeing the reality of our circumstances can put things in perspective. If nothing else, hopefully you'll see that feeling anxious, depressed, or stressed out and overwhelmed is not a personal failing. It is a predictable outcome of our long-outdated evolutionary wiring trying to cope with the complex circumstances of life in the twenty-first century.

Becoming conscious of the forces and behaviors working against us is the first step in training our minds and rewiring our brains to flourish. Many of us are so accustomed to the modern way of doing things that we don't even realize we are battling ourselves. We didn't sign up for a continuous stream of news hijacking our brains or smartphones designed to keep us distracted, scattered, and disconnected from actual human contact. We are all participants in a grand experiment for which we didn't give our informed consent. None of us are immune. From climate change, political polarization, and global warfare on the one hand to raising children and caring for aging parents on the other, the stress of modernity affects all walks of life.

Constant worry and stress erode our mental health and, by extension, our physical health. Despite the great technological and medical advances in modern society, life expectancy is declining for the first time in history for parts of the population in many developed countries, including the United States. Angus Deaton, the Nobel Prize–winning economist at Princeton, has described this premature mortality as "deaths of despair," since many of these deaths are suicides, drug overdoses, and other tragedies tied to our declining mental health.

So, the question arises: Why is it important to know about what is happening around us? Doesn't all the bad news only make things worse? In fact, as we'll discuss in chapter 5, awareness is the necessary prerequisite for change. To pull ourselves out of these depths and get on the path to flourishing, it's helpful to understand how all these outside factors affect us and cause us to behave. If we're not aware of the forces surrounding us, it's difficult to loosen their grip on our minds and bodies. A line of research at the Center for Healthy Minds strongly supports the idea that when we're not aware of the factors influencing us, it's very difficult to regulate our responses. But when we're aware, change becomes possible. So, from the barrage of news to smartphone addiction, identifying and examining how these influences affect us is where we begin our journey to flourishing. We cannot change what we're not aware of.

There's another reason why awareness of these negative influences is important: the facts about them are often less of an obstacle than the myths we believe about them. For example, some might say they can't flourish because of their genetics, while others will argue they can't because they don't earn enough money. We will show you that such constraints on flourishing are often less significant than we think. It's easy to buy into the stories we tell ourselves, so discerning between fact and myth will help to provide the confidence that we can flourish despite our circumstances.

Let's look at some of the more prominent obstacles to our flourishing. Admittedly, there are many we do not consider here, including climate change, illness, work stress, and family stress, but we do consider a few of the obstacles that are universally challenging in today's world.

The Digital World

Look at people standing in line to get their morning coffee or waiting to board a plane at the airport. Whenever there is a moment of downtime, out comes the smartphone. We seem unable to resist the seductive lure of our digital devices. There is now a growing scientific literature on smartphone addiction, with some findings even showing abnormalities in brain regions found with other forms of addiction. Hundreds of studies show that a dopamine-rich part of the brain called the ventral striatum, which is involved in reward and motivation, is abnormally activated in drug addiction. Smartphone addiction operates on this same circuit. We've become so attached to our devices that many people feel anxious if they haven't checked their messages or switched on their phones after as little as ten minutes.

Such extreme smartphone addiction is associated with an increased likelihood of anxiety and depression. Researchers have seen improved mental health outcomes in recent studies where participants have limited their smartphone usage. For example, in a recent study from Germany, 500 adult participants were asked to reduce their smartphone use by 60 minutes daily for 14 days. After the 14-day period, participants were free to use their smartphone as much or as little as they wished. Those who had been assigned to the group instructed to reduce their smartphone use by 60 minutes voluntarily maintained their reduction over a 3-month period. In fact, they actually showed a small further reduction in use over this period. Three months later, at a follow-up, the researchers noted a 30 percent reduction in depressive symptoms. These and other related findings clearly indicate that the pervasive overuse of smartphones is contributing to the global deterioration in our flourishing.

It's important to recognize that this isn't a black-and-white scenario. Some device use can improve our social connection. There are several clear benefits to the technology we've all been provided. Still, it certainly can be difficult to put down our devices, and the struggle to moderate our device usage is a universal one.

The Cost of Distraction

Have you ever crawled into bed after a stressful day, reached for your phone to set your morning alarm, and then found a new message that grabbed your attention? Soon enough, you've clicked a few links, and you're scrolling through news feeds, articles, and videos that you never intended to read or watch in the first place. Before you know it, you've spent an hour of your life taking in a mind-numbing barrage of information. You wanted to relax, unwind, and get some rest, but instead, you're now feeling scattered and unfulfilled.

In the modern world, the pull of distraction is everywhere. When you begin the rewarding journey of cultivating awareness, you will notice this constant pull of distraction. You are not alone. Around the same time Richie was researching pain with meditators, another research team was doing some groundbreaking work on distraction. Matt Killingsworth and Dan Gilbert, two psychologists from Harvard, were using an innovative method called "experience sampling" to see how distracted people are in daily life. They sent smartphone notifications to more than 2,000 research subjects, asking them throughout the day what they were doing, whether they were aware and paying attention, and how they felt. The results were striking.

They found that the typical person is distracted *nearly half of their waking life* (46.9 percent, to be exact). This was true during a wide range of activities, from boring activities like commuting to pleasant experiences like a nice conversation. They also found that people are less happy when thinking about other things. You would expect people to be less happy when distracted from positive experiences. Who wants to be distracted during something pleasant, right? But it turns out that people are also less happy when they're distracted versus not distracted in unpleasant situations as well.

Imagine you're starting your day with an overwhelming number of things to get done. You are scattered, distracted, and "up in your head" obsessing about your to-do list. You might get caught up in the endless inner commentary and have less mental and emotional energy for whatever you're doing in the moment. You might not notice your cute pet staring up at you for breakfast. Simply put, a scattered and distracted state doesn't feel good and will probably cause more stress.

Being present feels completely different. Summarizing the takeaway from their research, Killingsworth and Gilbert wrote: "A human mind is a wandering mind, and a wandering mind is an unhappy mind. The ability to think about what is not happening is a cognitive achievement that comes at an emotional cost." In short, distraction is toxic. It can ruin a moment of genuine human connection, undermine a productive stream of work or a moment of creative insight, and even make a challenging moment more challenging.

These days, the biggest source of distraction is that little device we carry in our pockets. If you're like the average person, you look at your phone about 150 times a day. But how many of those times do you look at it consciously and intentionally? How many apps do you open with intention? When you find yourself doomscrolling in bed or checking your messages when you should be working, are you doing it on purpose?

Many of us lose our motivation to keep practicing regulation when we see how distracted we are. When we sit down to do an awareness practice, we face how challenging it is to follow a simple instruction like paying attention to our breath. Our minds wander all over the place like a restless monkey jumping from tree to tree. Everyone gets distracted. It's a universal experience. If you sit down to meditate with a hundred other people, they might look calm and serene on the outside, but everyone is struggling with restlessness and distraction. The importance of consciously regulating our impulses has never been greater.

PRACTICE

Distraction Reflection

Simply noticing that you are distracted is the first step in cultivating awareness. If you keep it up, these brief moments of recognizing distraction slowly become lasting experiences of focus, presence, and inner calm.

Take some time now to explore your habits of distraction by reflecting on each of the following questions. It can be helpful to write down your responses.

What are your go-to sources of distraction? Do you binge-watch your favorite shows? Get caught up in social media? Do you eat, drink, or use some other substance? What is your main way to escape the present moment?

What situations or experiences do you most commonly distract yourself from? Are there specific feelings or emotions you try to avoid? Are there situations or memories you commonly find yourself distracted by? Try to remain open and curious as you reflect on your experiences with distraction.

Imagine your life if you were less distracted. Think of specific activities and relationships that are important to you and how they might change if you brought more awareness to them. What would it be like to live with more awareness at these times?

Social Isolation

Richie is the director of the Center for Healthy Minds, where more than sixty people are on staff. He found only five people working at the Center on a Thursday afternoon in November. Where have all the people gone? Since Covid, things have shifted. Although so many people feel socially isolated these days, many still choose to work remotely if they can. This is an ongoing challenge for Richie in his role as director. On the one hand, he wishes to respect the staff's preferences; on the other, more in-person connections would benefit many of us at this time.

During the writing of this book, the then–US surgeon general, Dr. Vivek H. Murthy, issued a health advisory about the current crisis in our mental health as a nation. Presenting sobering evidence for significant downward trends in social connection and significant upward trends in loneliness and social isolation, Dr. Murthy emphasized that we aren't just more stressed than ever—we are also more alone than ever. Most of us are spending an average of 24 more hours a month alone than we were 15 years ago. What's more, most of us are spending 20 fewer hours a month socializing with our friends. We (Richie and Cort) are no different. Sometimes we find ourselves randomly scrolling through the news rather than spending that time with family.

Social isolation exacts an enormous cost on our health. Loneliness is not simply a subjective emotional state—it gets under our skin and causes premature mortality. In fact, the surgeon general noted that loneliness is a greater-than-twofold risk factor for dying early compared to obesity.

Our behavior also changes due to social isolation, and that has an impact on the many different systems in the brain. For example, we know that loneliness impairs decision-making and is associated with reduced gray matter volume in the brain's prefrontal cortex, a key region responsible for planning and decision-making. Our prefrontal cortex is constantly making predictions about the world and refining these predictions based on feedback from our experiences. When we're socially isolated, we're deprived of regular feedback from others. We depend upon this feedback for calibration and to increase the accuracy of our predictions about the world. So, when we're socially deprived or feel alone, we're literally less able to read the world accurately.

Loneliness is often accompanied by social anxiety and the tendency to perceive others, particularly those outside our immediate in-group, as potential threats. The faces of strangers then activate the fear circuitry in the brain, and our perception of others reflects this bias.

Social isolation also compromises our insula, the brain region involved in empathy and compassion. As we noted in chapter 2, it is the only brain region that has a topographic map of the different visceral organs in the body. A key node in mind-brain-body interaction, the insula literally engages the body to enable us to feel what others are experiencing. So when we feel lonely, our insula takes a hit, making it even harder for us to feel connected to others.

Beyond Our Control?

Flourishing can seem daunting in the face of all the obstacles we face, and many seem beyond our control. Maybe you're asking yourself if it's even possible to flourish. For example, how can we possibly flourish when we are barraged with bad news? What if we're struggling to make ends meet? What if we're convinced we just don't have the right genetics to flourish? And what about trauma? So many of us have faced some type of trauma, which can feel impossible to overcome.

These are just a few of the many factors beyond our control that challenge our flourishing. For any given person, there are likely many more, from sickness to the need to provide long-term care for a loved one to facing natural disasters, to name just a few. We want to highlight the four most common challenges: the twenty-four-hour news cycle, money, trauma, and genetics. Each is also fraught with widespread misconceptions, especially in relation to flourishing.

First, it's important we consider the actual evidence for how these factors can influence flourishing. Then, we need to ask how much influence they really have. By reviewing the evidence, we hope to show you that these four common obstacles are not nearly as formidable as they seem. And once you begin to cultivate the skills we teach in later chapters, you will find that you can still train yourself to flourish.

The Twenty-Four-Hour News Cycle

The barrage of information about the very real threats of hyperpolarization, systemic injustice, devastating global conflicts, and climate change all profoundly impact our ability to flourish. Research evidence clearly documents that the more exposure we have to the news in general, the more anxiety and depression we experience. In a study with about 450 participants, the more they doomscrolled, the less life satisfaction, psychological well-being, and relationship harmony they reported.

How can we flourish if we're constantly on alert? We could spend an entire book covering all the evidence on how exposure to negative news impairs our flourishing. Racism and systemic injustice have been linked to abnormal hyperactivity of the brain's threat circuitry, including the amygdala, a key structure in the detection of threat. While the impact these challenges have on the brain has been studied in isolation, the synergistic impact of all of them operating together has not been studied but likely erodes the brain's functioning in devastating ways. The combination of these elements creates a perfect storm that arouses our threat and fear circuits and poses challenges to our capacity to flourish.

Flourishing doesn't make the world's problems go away, but it does provide us with the skills to cope. Given the news we are faced with in our world, feeling stressed, anxious, and depressed is only human—you are not alone. But flourishing is also human, and we can train ourselves to flourish more and stress less. Because we are born to flourish, our pre-wiring makes it possible to shift our state of mind and behaviors toward flourishing. Simple, but maybe not easy—especially when people believe their flourishing is fixed by factors over which they have little or no control.

Money

Western culture seems predicated on the assumption that more money equals more happiness, which equals more flourishing. Capitalist society is oriented toward continual growth. If you examine a graph that depicts the trend line for Gross Domestic Product, or GDP (a summary metric of all the goods and services purchased within a unit of time), you would see that for the past fifty years, this number has been steadily trending upward in the United States and most economically developed countries. But a graph that plots the average well-being of the US over the same time period would show a line with a downward trend. This is just one of many data points that leads us to question whether money and flourishing go hand in hand.

The relationship between money and flourishing has been debated for hundreds of years. Most commentators in modern psychology over the past hundred years acknowledge the critical importance of money for our health and well-being. In Abraham Maslow's famous hierarchy of needs, after basic physiological needs, our greatest needs are safety and security, both of which are significantly influenced by money. You could argue that many factors subsumed within the first rung of physiological needs—such as shelter, clothing, and even sleep—depend upon money. If we cannot rest in a safe and quiet place, our capacity to sleep will be significantly impaired. Sadly, millions of people today do not have safe and quiet places to sleep.

Shigehiro Oishi, a cross-cultural psychologist and highly creative researcher, has studied the relationship between money and flourishing in novel ways. He began his work by acknowledging, as most scholars do, that there is some relationship between money and flourishing. He then asked whether flourishing continues to increase indefinitely as income rises. Is Elon Musk (putatively the wealthiest person in the world) flourishing significantly more than, say, LeBron James, who is worth $1 billion? Musk is at least one hundred times wealthier than James. Is Musk's flourishing one hundred times greater? We think even common sense dissuades us from believing that flourishing scales linearly with wealth.

Oishi set out to determine empirically whether there are "income satiation" points beyond which increases in wealth do not impact flourishing. He was also interested in discovering whether there might be what he called "turning points" where further increases in wealth result in declines in flourishing. To answer these questions, Oishi and his colleagues used sophisticated statistical methods to identify points of income satiation in data from the Gallup World Poll that contained a representative sample of 1.7 million individuals systematically sampled from every region of the world. Using measures of emotional well-being as the key target—similar to what we would define as flourishing—Oishi and his colleagues learned that satiation occurs globally with an annual income between $60,000 to $75,000. Increases past $75,000 have no additional benefit for our flourishing.

Not surprisingly, there was considerable variation in different parts of the world, with satiation occurring later in richer countries. The satiation point in North America (the US and Canada) was between $65,000 and $95,000.

The important point of this research is that, yes, money does matter, but only up to a point. Beyond that, not only does it not predict increases in flourishing, but in many parts of the world, higher income levels are associated with a "turning point" where flourishing actually begins to decline.

During a visit to Bhutan, Richie was walking in a fairly remote part of the country with his friend Matthieu Ricard, a French Buddhist monk who has spent many years living there. They encountered a nomad on the trail walking to a village where he was going to attend a festival. Richie asked him how long he had been walking; he said for four days. He was dressed in rags, and although he carried few possessions, he radiated joy and seemed to be flourishing. This man probably earned less than $5,000 a year, yet he offered us some biscuits from his backpack. Clearly, in some cases, we can flourish even if we are way short of the saturation point.

There is another way in which money influences our flourishing. Imagine how a schoolteacher would feel if they received a 10 percent increase in their salary. Now imagine how this same teacher would feel if after being informed of this 10 percent increase, their colleague in the same school received a 20 percent raise. A wealth of evidence shows that perceived income inequality is detrimental to our flourishing. In most instances, rather than being happy for our colleague's big raise, we feel sorry for ourselves. Even though we might be perfectly happy with our salary, we now somehow feel less valued in a more personal way.

Social comparison is a difficult challenge to our flourishing, yet it is so deeply embedded within Western culture. But we can learn to defuse the toxic emotions that might arise from it and harness this energy to fuel the vitality that is needed for systemic change. In the longer term, both individual and systemic change are necessary and synergistic. Together, they can lead to enduring social transformation.

Money clearly has some effect on flourishing. However, both our experience and the evidence show that while it sets some broad constraints on how much flourishing is possible, we can still learn simple skills to improve our ability to navigate adversity even in very difficult circumstances.

Trauma

We would be remiss if we failed to recognize the powerful impact trauma has on our ability to flourish and on the biology that supports our flourishing. Our colleague Jamie Hanson has led much of the work on trauma at the Center for Healthy Minds. The primary purpose of our initial work on this topic was to document the impact of early trauma on children's brain development. Jamie recruited, via their parents, 128 12-year-old kids who had experienced various kinds of adversity and trauma in their early life, including emotional abuse (some were orphaned or abandoned), physical abuse, and poverty. We also had a control group of kids the same age who did not experience any form of early adversity.

The abused children were internationally adopted from institutions for orphaned or abandoned children in Romania. They had spent an average of 30 months in institutional care before they were adopted and were a little over 3 years old when they were welcomed into middle-class homes in the United States.

We performed brain (MRI) scans on the 12-year-olds to measure the size of different subregions of their brains, particularly structures important for emotion and emotion regulation. What we found was powerful and distressing. Compared with the control children, the ones who experienced early-life trauma had a smaller hippocampus and amygdala—critical structures for emotion and emotion regulation—making it harder for these kids to adopt the skills necessary for flourishing.

Because we had detailed life histories from the adoptive parents of each child's cumulative lifetime exposure to stress and trauma, we were able to identify that the earlier stress and trauma had occurred in a child's life, the smaller their amygdala and hippocampus. As we noted earlier in this chapter, adversity truly "gets under the skin," affecting the brain in profound ways that impair the ability to flourish.

What is trauma exactly? And what does this mean for all of us? Trauma ultimately is our subjective interpretation of adversity. Many of us are impacted by trauma in both large and small cumulative ways. In a very important study published in 2020, Andrea Danese of the Institute of Psychiatry at King's College in London and his colleague Cathy Widom at John Jay College of Criminal Justice of the City University of New York studied 1,196 adults. They were given questionnaires asking them about maltreatment and abuse when they were children. And what is most important in this study is that objective, court-documented records of maltreatment were available in this group from when they were children. Their findings revealed something dramatic. Even in cases of severe childhood maltreatment identified through court records, the risk of psychiatric disorder was minimal unless there was an accompanying subjective report of trauma when they were adults. If there was a subjective report of trauma, even in the absence of any objective court-documented maltreatment, the risk of psychiatric disorder was equally high as the group with both objective and subjective evidence of trauma. In other words, what matters is our subjective experience.

The fact that significant maltreatment can occur without leading to a reaction of trauma and subsequent mental health problems is good news for plasticity. In our own work with teenagers from Colombia who experienced extreme abuse as infants and children, we found that an intensive intervention to promote flourishing skills had a dramatic impact on their ability to heal. In this study, 44 teenage girls with more than 5 significant adverse childhood experiences were randomized to an intensive week of flourishing intervention or treatment as usual. After the flourishing intervention, there was a 76 percent decline in symptoms compared with a 17 percent decline in the treatment-as-usual group. These changes remained stable at a 2-month follow-up. In these same teenagers, we found the flourishing program induced epigenetic changes, with alterations in the expression of genes associated with inflammation, cancer, cardiovascular disease, and brain plasticity itself. These findings are a proof of concept that even with very significant trauma, we can heal.

Genetics

One of the common methods used to figure out whether a behavioral trait is influenced by heritable genetic factors is with a study comparing fraternal and identical twins. Identical twins share all their genes; this is what makes them identical. Fraternal twins share half their genes; they are as genetically related to each other as any two siblings from the same mother and father. We measure a particular trait or variable to see whether or not it is heritable and compare the correlation between the two members of the twin pair (co-twins). If the correlation between the identical co-twins is significantly higher than the correlation between the fraternal co-twins, it's evidence for heritability.

What do heritability studies say about our ability to flourish?

When this procedure is followed for measures of well-being and flourishing, genetic effects account for somewhere between 40 and 50 percent of the magnitude of flourishing. Said a different way, about half of what determines our level of flourishing is produced by genetic factors. There is indeed a clear genetic influence on flourishing, but there is also still a lot of room for other influences, such as the many skills and practices we'll explore in later chapters.

So what do we make of the fact that 40 to 50 percent of the variation among people in their levels of flourishing is due to genetic factors? How should we interpret this? How much is our level of flourishing dictated by our genes? Clearly, we take a different position in suggesting that well-being can be cultivated. But how much does our genetic makeup constrain how much we can improve?

Michael Meaney is a scientist who studies epigenetics at McGill University in Montreal, Canada. A brilliant and provocative thinker, Michael is one of Richie's scientific heroes. Early in his career, Meaney's work with animals provided some of the most important evidence for epigenetic changes in response to experience. Remember from chapter 2 that epigenetics is the science of how our genes are regulated and that they have little volume controls that can be turned up or down to regulate how much of the protein they're designed to manufacture actually gets produced.

A number of years ago, Richie invited Michael to be part of a small group of scientists traveling to Dharamsala, India, to meet with the Dalai Lama to brief him on the latest advances in science. Richie thought Michael's work would be especially interesting and relevant because it is among the most powerful bodies of evidence to show that experience and training can dramatically alter our biology. It is this work that leads us to question the nature/nurture question itself. Let us explain.

Anxiety is a trait that is at least partially heritable. When scientists work with rats, they can selectively breed them by pairing a highly anxious male and a highly anxious female and then take their offspring and pair them with the offspring of another highly anxious pairing, and so on for many generations. Because rats have much shorter life spans (about three years) than people, scientists can selectively breed many generations fairly quickly. What we end up with after several generations of in-breeding for high-anxious traits and low-anxious traits are two groups of rats that are dramatically different in behavior. The highly anxious rats are very scared of new environments. They are hypervigilant and often freeze, their appetite is suppressed, and their heart rates are elevated. Low-anxious rats are just the opposite. They explore new environments, eat normally, move around a lot, and their heart rates are low.

After he bred rats this way for several generations, Michael did an experiment that one obviously couldn't do on humans. He cross-fostered the young rats from the high- and low-anxious groups. Specifically, the high-anxious rat pups were raised by low-anxious, laid-back mothers, and vice versa. If genes control our behavior, then the differential rearing of cross-fostering should make little difference. On the other hand, if epigenetic factors are at play, then maybe the biology of the highly anxious rat pups could be modified by their exposure to the laid-back rat moms. Guess what happened?

The results strongly support the epigenetic hypothesis. The highly anxious rat pups raised by laid-back mothers became dramatically less anxious. The environment, in this case, was the most important determinant. You can think of this as immersion exposure since the rat pups were exposed to their cross-fostered mothers from birth. When Michael analyzed the epigenetics of the highly anxious rat pups after their exposure to laid-back mothers, he found the genes coding for anxiety were down-regulated. There were also systematic changes in the rat pups' brains. Thus, the rearing behaviors of the laid-back rat mothers got "under the skin," dramatically impacting gene expression and altering brain function and structure.

Because of findings like this, we cannot adjudicate between nature and nurture. It is always both. But what the Michael Meaney findings show is that experientially induced epigenetic effects can be very powerful and enough to overcome a strong genetic bias. This is a hugely important insight because it means that even though there is some genetic basis that partially explains why some people flourish more than others, it really has no bearing on a person's capacity to learn to flourish more. Simply because a psychological trait has some genetic contribution says nothing about its modifiability.

Flourishing in the Face of Adversity

The take-home message here is that although life in the twenty-first century is filled with challenges, flourishing is possible. Your genetic heritage will not determine the course your life will take, nor will a major life trauma, your income, or any other external circumstance. All these factors play a role in shaping your ability to flourish, but there are many other factors that matter as well—and some of the most important, including the ones that form the heart of this book, are innate capacities that you can recognize and nurture through practice.

Flourishing is thus much more than happiness. You won't feel happy if you lose your job or find yourself struggling with a major health issue, but, as strange as it may sound, you can flourish in difficult periods. You can use any moment of life—positive, negative, and anything in between—as an opportunity to nurture the most meaningful and fulfilling aspects of your life.

This is precisely what started Cort on his personal journey as a college student in the early 1990s. Cort was always a little anxious as a teenager, but his stress levels went through the roof when he stepped onto campus for the first time and found himself thrown into the deep end of college life. Making new friends, staying on top of his classes, the pressure of trying to "find himself" and figure out what he wanted to do with his life—it was all too much. He was completely overwhelmed.

Cort's sky-high levels of anxiety were crippling at times. He stopped going out with his friends. His schoolwork suffered, and by the end of his first semester, he had to drop one class and was getting close to dropping out altogether. He felt like he'd made a complete mess of his life. Everything seemed to be spiraling out of control.

But the mess was only part of the story.

The feeling of an impending catastrophe spurred Cort to look for a way out, and the most painful period of his life eventually became the most fulfilling. It was certainly not a joyful period by any stretch of the imagination, but it was a time of intense introspection and self-discovery. He started a regular meditation practice and discovered new ideas that completely changed his outlook on life and his views of himself and his own potential. He was, in a sense, flourishing. His struggles opened the door to possibilities that never would have happened if he'd been happy and content.

You may not struggle with anxiety like Cort did, but chances are you have struggled with something. Every one of us grapples with inner demons. Every one of us will face difficulties in our lives, from the loss of loved ones to health problems to work stress. There is no version of human life that does not involve pain and suffering, and simply hoping that we can avoid all these problems is unrealistic. The wise course of action is to equip yourself so you can flourish in the midst of adversity.

Chances are that some part of you already knows how to do this. Think back on your life. Can you think of a time of loss or grief that propelled you to experience deep love and connection to those around you? Or perhaps a major life challenge connected you to a strong sense of purpose and a heightened awareness of the preciousness of human life. These experiences are more common than you might think.

In the next few chapters, you'll be introduced to the path to flourishing. We'll share simple strategies for each skill to help you strengthen that skill gradually over time. You will become more aware, more connected, more insightful, and more purposeful with simple practices that you can sprinkle throughout your day. We will show you that even five minutes a day of intentionally training your mind can help you tap your full potential to flourish.

Chapter 4

The Path to Flourishing

> What you are looking for is already in you . . . You already are everything you are seeking.
>
> —Thich Nhat Hanh

One of the most challenging periods of Richie's life occurred when his son, Seth, was in high school. As a three-week-old infant, Seth suffered a severe case of meningitis that produced seizures and landed him in the hospital for a ten-day stay. Richie and his wife, Susan, almost lost him. Years later, they discovered that the meningitis had left scarring in the parietal lobe of Seth's brain, an area important for integrating sensory information and creating links between different modes of experience, like the connection between a visual symbol and what it represents, which showed up as struggles with learning.

As a freshman in high school, for example, Seth was required to memorize the different parts of a male and female flower—the anther, filament, stigma, and petals. The preferred and most helpful strategy for memorizing such material is to visualize the flower and then link the labels to the different parts. This cognitive maneuver requires an intact parietal cortex and was precisely the kind of task Seth struggled with. Today, this would be a textbook case of neurodivergence. It was also an early warning sign that something was a little different about Seth compared to his older sister, Amelie, who sailed through high school and graduated from a top-tier university.

Once Seth got to high school, he began to check out and experiment with drugs. As he grew even less interested in school, his academic problems grew worse, and the difficulties started to spiral. His teenage curiosity became more dangerous and destructive, and Seth's alienation at home and at school led to emotional pain and distress for the whole family, especially Seth.

Although Richie had decades of meditation experience, this life experience pushed him further than any before. Several things came into focus very quickly. The first was the narrative Richie had constructed in his mind about his children. While his daughter mostly conformed to this narrative, Seth did not. Richie became very curious about this narrative and how it was affecting his behavior. He saw how this traditional story about "success" filtered his worldview, and the distortion and pain it caused came sharply into focus. Richie and his wife's purpose in this major life event also became apparent. Richie's shifted from trying to fix the situation to simply loving his son. This shift had a profound effect on the entire family system. While acutely painful, the episode brought Richie's family much closer together. Although Richie was not happy about what was transpiring, he flourished. Seth ended up becoming a school psychologist, happily married, and the wonderful father of two beautiful boys.

Meetings with Remarkable People

Richie's experience as a parent carried an important lesson: we *can* weather the big storms of life, but we need to tap into our inner skills and resources to do so. When we do, we can flourish even when facing an unexpected setback, a major loss, or a health challenge.

In 2012, years after Richie's experience with his son, Cort moved to Madison to begin his doctoral work. We immediately began a deep dialogue about the nature of flourishing. The first thing we set out to do was to establish a solid definition. As we shared our personal histories, we noticed that we had both experienced flourishing in the face of hardship. These weren't memories of happiness or joy but rather of learning important lessons about life and the human condition in the midst of adversity. It was clear to both of us that flourishing looked different in different circumstances, but when we asked ourselves why we flourished in some situations but felt overwhelmed in others, we couldn't quite put our fingers on it. The actual building blocks of flourishing weren't so clear.

Modern science has a lot to say about the nature of human flourishing. Scientists have been studying well-being and presenting different models of it for decades. The two most influential models focus on "hedonic" and "eudaimonic" well-being. This way of thinking about flourishing has roots in the philosophy of Aristotle, who wrote about *hedonia* as the experience of pleasure and *eudaimonia* as the pursuit of meaning, purpose, and self-actualization. Drawing on Aristotle's insightful distinction, scientists formed different models of human flourishing, some more focused on hedonic elements of well-being, such as positive emotions, and others on eudaimonic aspects, including personal growth and life purpose.

After exploring different ideas about flourishing, we got curious about training. Could we train ourselves to flourish? We had deep discussions about the various meditation traditions with their detailed descriptions of the emotional and psychological qualities that lead to states of flourishing and their clear road maps for training those qualities. In the Tibetan tradition, for instance, there is a path of meditative self-exploration known as Mahamudra. In this approach, you turn awareness toward itself. Instead of focusing on a meditative object like the breath, the emphasis is on the knowing quality of the mind. You first learn to recognize the presence of awareness and then explore this knowing, subjective quality of experience. This process of inner exploration is said to lead to transformative insights into the very nature of human consciousness. The Mahamudra teachings are incredibly detailed, with step-by-step instructions for exploring and transforming the mind.

But where were such systems of training in modern science? They were nowhere to be found. We had pinpointed a major gap in the prevailing scientific models of flourishing and well-being. Most of the research done up to that point was correlational. For the most part, it looked at different aspects of well-being and how they relate to things like health outcomes and other variables, but it didn't have much to say on the topic of training. Can the core dimensions of flourishing be strengthened? If so, how? What are the most effective strategies for doing so? Research on training well-being and cultivating states of flourishing was largely absent.

We were mystified. Why would there be such a glaring hole in the research literature, especially on such an obviously important topic? There was a growing body of research in the study of mindfulness and a little bit in positive psychology, but science had barely scratched the surface of practice and training. It was pretty new territory.

The absence created an opportunity. As we pondered how we might study the cultivation of flourishing, our conversation turned to the remarkable people we'd met over the years. Richie had studied some of the world's most advanced meditators, Tibetan Buddhist monks. His thinking had been that if he could find some data that distinguished their experiences, he could compare them with less advanced practitioners and eventually with novices to understand more about how contemplative practice affects the brain. On the other hand, if he couldn't find any meaningful changes in people who had practiced for tens of thousands of hours, there probably wouldn't be much hope of seeing signs of change in everyday meditators.

When Richie set out to study these "advanced meditators," he had so many questions: When we put them in the scanner, will their brains respond differently from those of other people? How will they respond to challenging situations, like physical pain or public speaking? Will they get worked up ahead of time or ruminate afterward—like the rest of us? He had no idea.

To get answers to these questions, Richie put them in all sorts of challenging situations. He examined how they responded to pain by observing the brain's pain matrix and comparing it to the brain activity of an adult non-meditator. He made them do complex math calculations and public-speaking exercises to elicit a stress reaction. And then there was the experience of putting them in the brain scanner. The monks agreed to spend hours and hours lying motionless in a freezing-cold room doing tedious cognitive tests that helped Richie's team of scientists see how an advanced meditator's brain functions differently from a non-meditator brain. These state-of-the-art fMRI brain scanners measured changes in the oxygenation of the blood in the monks' brains, which indirectly reflected which regions were more active during different forms of practice. He also covered their heads with EEG electrodes to measure their brains' electrical activity. Each subject spent days in the laboratory as Richie and his team took measurements.

This early research led to some of the most important findings in what was then a completely new field of scientific research. There was indeed something different about these advanced meditators—in some cases, dramatically different. But it wasn't just their brain activity and how their nervous systems responded to stress. The way they carried themselves seemed fundamentally different as well. They weren't like any other people Richie had ever met.

Richie spent countless hours with the Tibetan monks during his research. Although they spent long periods in brain scanners and days doing tedious tests over and over again, they remained in good spirits the entire time. Not only did Richie and the other scientists not need to care for the monks, but the reverse happened. The monks ended up taking care of them. If something went wrong in one of the experiments, the monks didn't get agitated as most people would. When Richie or any of the other scientists got worked up about something, the monks would do something to help. Occasionally, they'd lighten the mood with their playful sense of humor; at other moments, they offered reassuring words to calm everyone down. It was like they were having the time of their lives. The monks continued to flourish in a stressful lab experience, just as they did at home.

While Richie was conducting this pioneering research, Cort was living in Tibetan refugee settlements in Nepal and India. He became fluent in Tibetan, translating the ancient meditation manuals these same meditators used in their training. Cort also got to know these remarkable people. He did long meditation retreats under their guidance, spending countless hours learning about the practice of meditation and the intricacies of the human mind. After living with and among them for nearly a decade, Cort reached the same conclusion Richie had. These people were different. They seemed to embody an inner mastery he had never witnessed before. These were true masters of the art of training and transforming the mind.

As we shared everything we'd learned from our research and personal experience, we realized that if we wanted to better understand how to cultivate flourishing, the first place to look was at them. The monks seemed preternaturally joyful, funny, compassionate, and wise in almost any situation. Their joy was contagious, and even more, it was inspiring given the fact that they were all refugees living in refugee settlements in one of the poorest countries in Asia. These monks had almost nothing—no bank accounts, few belongings, and not many of the things most of us take for granted—and yet, they were clearly thriving.

As we continued to reflect on these remarkable people, we tried to pinpoint what made them so special. Some were celibate monks and nuns, while others had families and jobs. Some were quiet and introspective, but a few were gregarious and outgoing. Despite all the differences, there were some striking similarities. All seemed to be flourishing. But what were the qualities of flourishing exactly? We noted that the monks were always present and attentive in any given moment. They never seemed to be "somewhere else" or distracted. What's more, they were wise, filled with insights about the human condition, and they showed tremendous care and concern for the people around them. They radiated warmth and inner peace, and despite their seemingly carefree attitude, it was clear they were guided by a deep and abiding sense of purpose. They all seemed to share a commitment to bringing more wisdom and compassion into our troubled world.

We realized we did not need to look any further. These extraordinary people were telling us all we needed to know about the most important dimensions of human flourishing, and their systematic practices showed it could be trained. We hadn't yet formed our own framework to understand these dimensions, but they were coming into focus. And as we learned more, we started to see striking connections between the ancient lineages of practice that focus on qualities like awareness, compassion, and wisdom and the cutting-edge research Richie and other leading scientists were doing.

The Monk in the Scanner

Of all the yogis and meditators we got to know, one Buddhist monk stood out: Yongey Mingyur Rinpoche. Our work with Rinpoche—both Richie's research in the lab and Cort's meditating under his guidance in India and Nepal—helped us pinpoint the most important dimensions of flourishing and the many practices that can be used to strengthen them.

When each of us first met Mingyur Rinpoche, he was in his twenties and had already spent years of his life meditating in retreat. Despite his young age, he had mastered the ancient practices of his Tibetan spiritual heritage: practices to maintain a nearly effortless state of undistracted presence, practices for feeling deeply connected to all living creatures, practices to generate wisdom and insight through self-inquiry and self-exploration, and practices for imbuing even the most mundane chore with a vibrant sense of purpose. When we put him in the brain scanner, we saw patterns of brain activity never before observed. The combination of his being such an adept meditator at such a young age and his passionate interest in psychology and neuroscience made Rinpoche the perfect candidate for our research. It later turned out that some of the most remarkable scientific findings were based on scans of his brain.

Richie invited Mingyur Rinpoche, a confident meditation teacher with a growing community of students worldwide, to visit the University of Wisconsin–Madison to be a subject in some of the most important early research on meditation. Around the same time, Cort was living in Kathmandu, Nepal, where he was doing intensive meditation retreats each year and translating Buddhist meditation manuals into English under Rinpoche's guidance. Although we had yet to meet, Richie and Cort were both in deep dialogue with Rinpoche about the nature of human consciousness and how it can be transformed through meditation.

When Mingyur Rinpoche visited Madison, Richie put him in an fMRI brain scanner to observe his brain activity during meditation. As he lay motionless in the scanner, a small group of scientists huddled around a bank of computers in the next room, eager to see the results. They could see changes in blood flow in his brain in real time, but something else caught their attention: his eyes. Rinpoche's gaze was unwavering. His eyes did not move or blink for minutes on end. There was no watering or apparent discomfort, and his pupils were not dilating. It looked like he was in a state of suspended animation.

Scientists like Richie knew well that Rinpoche's steady gaze reflected a unique pattern of brain activity and a state of heightened concentration. When the mind moves, different brain regions light up in a dance of electrical activity, triggering subtle changes in the visual apparatus: the eyes blink, the pupils dilate, and minor shifts occur in the eyeballs themselves. These fluctuations are biomarkers of mental and neural activity. The fact that Rinpoche's gaze displayed so little movement suggested that something extraordinary was happening in his brain.

Indeed, it was.

Once Richie and his team crunched the data, it was clear that Rinpoche and the other advanced meditators had strengthened their awareness (one of the core dimensions of flourishing) to such a degree that they could willfully control their attention, emotional responses, and thought activity. It was also clear that their intensive, lifelong training had impacted basic biological functions like their spontaneous eyeblink rate—a phenomenon documented more than a decade later in a peer-reviewed scientific report. These meditators were masters of awareness and connection, which gave them the ability to enter states of deep concentration at will and activate feelings of deep connection (both key traits in flourishing) like they were flipping a switch. Their years of training had produced a level of inner mastery that had never before been observed with the tools of modern science.

Practice, Practice, Practice

Mingyur Rinpoche displayed peak levels of mental and emotional well-being. He was flourishing. Even his brain seemed to be operating at another level compared to the rest of us. As we got to know Rinpoche and learned more about his life, it became clear that he was not born a paragon of happiness and well-being. He had *learned* how to flourish. Rinpoche was living evidence that our capacity to flourish is not predetermined by our DNA or limited by our circumstances. It is a skill, and it can be strengthened with dedicated practice.

Mingyur Rinpoche experienced overwhelming panic attacks as a young child. His struggles with panic and anxiety, well documented in his best-selling book *The Joy of Living*, continued for years, even when he entered a strict three-year meditation retreat in his early teens. He eventually learned to apply his meditation practice to his challenging emotions, and his panic attacks vanished. For most of the next decade, he continued to immerse himself in the practice of meditation, spending twelve or more hours a day practicing in strict retreat for years on end.

The strict training undertaken by Mingyur Rinpoche, coupled with his experience dealing with panic disorder, resulted in a profound inner transformation. His mastery of awareness gave him a supernatural ability to focus and concentrate. He was kind and caring toward everyone he encountered and wise beyond his years. His training as a Buddhist monk gave him a clear set of values to live by, with the transcendent purpose of helping all beings to awaken as his personal North Star.

Mingyur Rinpoche picked up the skills we need to flourish at an early age and practiced them consistently and diligently, racking up more than 30,000 hours of meditation in just a few decades. Once he reached a level of mastery most of us can only imagine, he kept going. His intensive practice was not unlike the fanatic dedication of the world's greatest athletes, artists, and others who are masters of their craft. He was single-minded in his focus. He woke up early in the morning to practice and then did more meditation before bed. In retreat, he would often practice for twelve hours a day, sometimes more, for years on end. He even applied esoteric techniques to master the states of deep dreamless sleep and dreaming, the "luminosity meditation" and "dream yoga" of Tibetan Buddhism. When he wasn't on retreat or doing his usual daily meditation routine, he was teaching others how to meditate.

In 2011, Mingyur Rinpoche took things even further. He left his life as a best-selling author and rock star meditation teacher to spend four and a half years wandering in the Himalayas, a move that shocked his global following. He could have been jet-setting around the world. Instead, he dropped everything to live in caves and beg for his food all to further his meditative training. He almost died from food poisoning.

We were awed by Mingyur Rinpoche's personal journey. But it was more than that. His extreme training also produced profound changes in his brain activity that signaled a rare ability to flourish. In one study, for example, we compared a group of novice meditators to a small group of very advanced practitioners that included Mingyur Rinpoche. Not surprisingly, we found that the advanced meditators could concentrate for longer periods and resist the pull of distraction to a much greater degree. Compared with the control group of new meditators, the advanced meditators showed more activation in a range of attention-related brain regions. The novice meditators, on the other hand, showed more activation in regions linked to poor attentional skills. This is exactly what we expected to find.

However, things got more interesting when we looked at the brain activity *within* the group of advanced meditators. The activation patterns of the most experienced meditators looked strikingly different from those with less experience. Keep in mind that this was a group of super-advanced meditators. Even the least experienced meditator in this group had completed tens of thousands of hours of lifetime practice. Nevertheless, there were clear differences among them. In the less experienced advanced meditators, we saw more activation in the brain's attentional network, and the activation was sustained for longer periods of time than we saw in the novice meditators. In the most advanced meditators, however, we found just the opposite. After a brief burst of activity in the attention network, the brain quickly returned to baseline. If you didn't know any better, you would have no way of knowing that these meditators were in a state of deep concentration.

We had stumbled upon the neural correlates of attentional mastery—a key component of awareness, one of the most important dimensions of flourishing. This discovery pointed us in exciting new directions. These advanced meditators had harnessed the power of neuroplasticity and tapped more of their genetic potential than the scientific community thought possible. Still, we had studied only a tiny fraction of what they were telling us. We had gathered some impressive data on states of mindful awareness and focused attention, but mindfulness was just the beginning. The real practice, we learned, was to cultivate feelings of connection with all forms of life and gain deep insight into the very nature of consciousness. According to these advanced meditators, this potent combination of awareness, connection, and insight transforms the way we see the world, including the way we see ourselves, leading to deep and lasting states of flourishing.

Getting to know advanced meditators like Mingyur Rinpoche led us one step closer to a more precise understanding of the dimensions of flourishing and the road map to cultivating them. As you will learn later in this chapter, the qualities we were observing in these unusual research subjects were the very same qualities that would eventually become the basis for a new scientific framework focused on the cultivation of flourishing. We just didn't know it yet.

Training the Mind to Flourish

The more we heard from Mingyur Rinpoche about wisdom and compassion, the more we could see that we had just scratched the surface of the ways that all the different forms of practice can help us to flourish. The scientific community was laser-focused on mindfulness at the time, but these meditators were telling us that mindfulness is just one of many forms of meditation and that meditation is only one form of contemplative practice. Mingyur Rinpoche began to share more details about his meditation training and what a typical day of practice consists of. What he told us bore little resemblance to mindful breathing and other styles of practice many of us equate with meditation.

"When I meditate, my session includes many different steps. It usually starts with something like bodhichitta," he told us, referring to the "heart of awakening," in which one forms the motivation to meditate to help relieve the suffering of all sentient beings. "I always start by reflecting on my motivation and forming a compassionate motivation for my practice. Then, I rest in open awareness for a while. Open awareness is the practice of simply being. You don't have to do anything other than exist. There is no special state of mind to achieve when you rest in open awareness. Whatever is going on in your mind and body, you just let it happen. There is nothing to do other than be present. That's open awareness. After that, I might do any number of different techniques, depending on the kind of meditation I'm working on. I might go deeper into the cultivation of love and compassion, slowly expanding the circle of care until no being is left out, not even the tiniest insect."

Mingyur Rinpoche went on to explain even more practices. He told us about analytical meditations to cultivate wisdom. "There are forms of meditation like Dzogchen and Mahamudra where you explore consciousness itself," he said. "These practices can produce a profound shift in experience. The normal feeling of separateness between 'self' and 'other' drops away, and you get a glimpse of pure awareness. In my tradition, these are considered the most profound and transformative meditations."

Mingyur Rinpoche's story reflected what we heard from other advanced meditators and masters of the art of flourishing. It was clear that consistent daily practice was a habit they all shared. It was also clear that the training they followed was rich and complex. It wasn't all about mindfulness and attention. Even a single brief meditation session might touch upon a range of qualities, from mindful awareness to a deep sense of purpose, from self-inquiry to nurturing warm, caring connections.

In hearing Mingyur Rinpoche and other master meditators describe their daily practice, it dawned on us that training the mind is no different from the way we might train the body. Ideally, a person will incorporate cardio, stretching, and strength training into their routine. Each has a different effect on the body. If you lift weights and do nothing else, you'll be out of balance. Similarly, walking is better than doing nothing, but if you add some intense cardio and strength training, you'll be in better shape. The art of flourishing works the same way: the wise path involves training the mind in a variety of ways.

The Core Dimensions of Flourishing

Our research told us that the path to inner flourishing demands both steady practice and a comprehensive approach to training the mind, one focused on a range of different qualities, from mindful awareness to deep insight into the workings of the human mind. We immediately set out to map a path to flourishing that would be doable for a typical person in the modern world. We were filled with questions: What do the world's wisdom traditions tell us are the most important dimensions of flourishing? What does modern science have to say about these dimensions? Can these qualities be cultivated? If so, how? These questions guided us through long discussions and deep explorations of both meditative and scientific understandings of flourishing and how it can be cultivated.

Right away, we noticed many differences in the world's wisdom traditions, but four dimensions of flourishing also emerged: *awareness, connection, insight,* and *purpose.* We found numerous references to these four in the literature of diverse contemplative traditions, and we became even more excited once we connected the dots to modern science, including our own research. Strong empirical evidence across various disciplines—from cognitive and affective neuroscience to clinical psychology, well-being research, and positive psychology—suggested that awareness, connection, insight, and purpose are vital components of human flourishing. The world's meditative traditions added the unique perspective that these four qualities are not simply dimensions of flourishing but also skills we can learn and practice.

Awareness: The Skill of Being Present

The first skill of flourishing is awareness.

"When you train your mind," one of the monks we studied explained, "the first thing you do is build awareness and train your attention. If your mind is distracted all the time, forget about cultivating connection and insight. It's impossible. You have to start with awareness. It's the foundation for everything."

As we explored the topic of awareness more deeply, we discovered detailed pathways to train attention and strengthen awareness. Some forms of training focus on deep states of concentration. Others are geared toward effortless states of being, like the open awareness practice that Mingyur Rinpoche told us about. And while there are traditional meditations to cultivate awareness, meditation is not the only way to practice this skill. There are also movement practices like mindful walking, tai chi, and yoga that can help people ground their attention in the present moment. There are even traditional contemplative practices that use household chores and other daily activities to practice the skill of awareness. Awareness can be trained.

Connection: The Art of Healthy Relationships

The second skill of flourishing is connection. Scientific research on well-being has long focused on positive social interactions and strong relationships as a core element of psychological well-being. Our research with meditators reinforced this understanding and also showed us that feelings of connection can be strengthened by cultivating inner qualities like appreciation, kindness, and compassion and then gradually extending these qualities to more and more people and even other living creatures. One of our advanced meditators said, "Our practices help us to nurture a strong sense of connection with our friends and loved ones. We build on this by gradually extending our compassion to include many people and many other living creatures. Our goal is to expand our circle of connection until no one is left out."

Learning to widen our circle to feel a strong sense of connection with people we might usually not care for is possible, but it doesn't happen automatically. It takes training. Our genetic wiring has primed us to form groups and inner circles and to exclude others. For this reason, you have to nurture feelings of appreciation, kindness, and compassion for the people close to you and then gradually extend those feelings to others, even those with whom you might struggle. Eventually, everyone is included, and your sense of connection to the people you love and care for becomes even stronger.

As we reviewed research literature on positive social connections and surveyed a variety of wisdom traditions, we found many practices that strengthen our sense of connectedness. We started to see that although we don't usually think of things like kindness and compassion as skills, they are. We can practice gratitude and consciously cultivate appreciation.

In the eighth century, the Buddhist sage Shantideva wrote: "Be a lamp for those who seek light, a bed for those who seek rest, and a servant for all those in need."

Five centuries later, the poet Rumi, one of the most cherished masters of Islam's Sufi tradition, expressed a similar sentiment: "Be a lamp, or a lifeboat, or a ladder. Help someone's soul heal. Walk out of your house like a shepherd."

Rumi describes the path to flourishing as a process of deepening our love for ourselves, others, and the divine. Buddhism contains detailed instructions on generating caring emotions like love and compassion and then extending them until no living creature is left out. In the modern world, you'll find practices like gratitude journaling in positive psychology and loving-kindness meditations in secular meditation training. Our research backs this up: connection is the second cornerstone of human flourishing.

Insight: Exploring the Nature of the Self

The third skill of flourishing is insight. Insight helps us see things clearly, from our relationships and our work to our reactions and emotions. It helps us see the forest from the trees and recognize when we're getting stuck in dysfunctional ways of thinking or acting. It gives us a fresh perspective so we can let go of beliefs that aren't serving us anymore and stay open to new possibilities. Insight is one of the most important keys to learning and growth.

We can develop insight through self-inquiry and self-exploration. For example, you might explore your reactions and emotional patterns with curiosity or challenge yourself to see beyond your assumptions and expectations. At more advanced stages, you might examine your very sense of self and come to see that who and what you are is infinitely richer and more complex than you might otherwise believe.

Insight into your own mind and how it works naturally leads to wisdom. What it means to be wise varies across traditions, as do the paths to cultivating insight, but there is broad agreement that inquiring into the nature of the mind and gaining insight into the nature of reality is deeply transformative. In a classic of meditative literature, *The Way of a Pilgrim*, a book from the Russian Orthodox Christian tradition, the anonymous author wrote: "The trouble is that we live far from ourselves and have but little wish to get any nearer to ourselves. Indeed, we are running away all the time to avoid coming face to face with our real selves, and we barter the truth for trifles."

This passage mirrors countless teachings from different meditative and spiritual traditions on the nature of the self and its relationship to suffering. Some traditions hold that our culture, upbringing, and personal histories can leave us with a distorted sense of self. The rigid beliefs we hold about ourselves create unhealthy emotional habits and thought patterns, which, in turn, lead to chronic stress and more intense forms of suffering. Self-inquiry, contemplation, and reflection can produce insight into these unhealthy patterns, replacing distorted beliefs and interpretations with wisdom and self-discovery.

Purpose: Finding Your True North

The fourth and final skill of flourishing is purpose. When we looked closely at the advanced meditators in our lab, all of whom exhibited high levels of flourishing, they rarely spoke about the quality of their attention or even the great insights they'd developed through their practice. Instead, they spoke about their personal journeys as part of something much larger than their personal fulfillment. In most cases, their own well-being seemed to be an afterthought. They were focused on a much larger vision: the awakening of all beings.

The importance of having a guiding sense of purpose in life is nothing new. There are entire websites dedicated to inspiring quotes, like the following one from Helen Keller: "Many persons have a wrong idea of what constitutes true happiness. It is not attained through self-gratification but through fidelity to a worthy purpose."

Not everyone agrees on what constitutes a worthy purpose, but there is broad consensus that focusing on a goal or aspiration beyond personal happiness is central to a rich and fulfilling life.

When we spoke to people who seemed to have a clear sense of purpose in life, it became clear that purpose is a skill. They had trained themselves to feel a sense of direction in life. Take this piece of advice from His Holiness the Dalai Lama: "Every day, think as you wake up: today I am fortunate to be alive. I have a precious human life. I am not going to waste it. I am going to use all my energies to develop myself, to expand my heart out to others, to achieve enlightenment for the benefit of all beings."

This is more than an empty platitude. The Dalai Lama is describing a practice. He spends hours every single day cultivating this altruistic mindset, and for those of us who don't have hours to spare, we share practical tips that even the busiest person can use to have more purpose and meaning in their lives.

A Framework for Flourishing

As we pulled the pieces together, a compelling scientific narrative took shape. Strong data showed that each of the four skills plays a critical role in our mental, emotional, and physical health. The fact that the evidence came from different fields made the case even stronger. We reviewed studies from cognitive, affective, and social neuroscience, from clinical and social psychology, from well-being research and positive psychology, and from large-scale epidemiological health research. We found evidence that the four dimensions can be strengthened through training, as well as emerging evidence of the brain networks and biological mechanisms that are harnessed when we train them.

Some of the most surprising blind spots were in the field of well-being research. When we reviewed the most widely studied theories of well-being, for instance, we found ample evidence for two of our four dimensions: connection and purpose. Both appeared in virtually every theory and framework we looked at. Awareness and insight, on the other hand, were nowhere to be found. Even though both empirical research and the world's wisdom traditions agree on their importance, awareness and insight were not even on the radar for the most influential scientists studying well-being. For example, there are thousands of studies on attentional networks in the brain, but comparatively few show how awareness and attention are central to mental health and emotional well-being. Similarly, there is a mountain of data showing how purpose helps us flourish, but almost nothing on how a sense of purpose is reflected in brain activity or how it can be strengthened.

Another surprising blind spot concerned the trainability of the four dimensions. Most of the research in this area focused on drawing correlations between well-being and other factors like physical health or work performance. Very few data in the field of well-being research focused on learning and cultivation. In other fields, by contrast, there was tons of data. The emerging field of mindfulness research, for example, was filled with data showing not only that present-centered awareness is a key component of flourishing but also that it can be easily trained.

The further we got, the more confident we became that the field of well-being research desperately needed a clear, simple framework to describe the most important skills of flourishing and how they can be cultivated. The Healthy Minds Framework was thus born. We introduced our new framework to the wider scientific community with a publication in the prestigious *Proceedings of the National Academy of Sciences* in 2020.

PRACTICE

The Healthy Minds Index

Shortly after we published the Healthy Minds Framework, we started working on a scientific tool to measure the four skills of awareness, connection, insight, and purpose—the Healthy Minds Index—and published it in a peer-reviewed scientific journal. We use this index in our research, but you can use it to set your personal baseline and measure how awareness, connection, insight, and purpose change over time. This will give you a sense of your strong areas and those with the most room for growth. The questions in the index might get you thinking about your life a little differently. If nothing else, they'll give you a sense of how we think about the four skills and try to measure them.

To measure your current levels of the four skills, answer and score the following questions from the index.

HEALTHY MINDS INDEX

All items are rated on a 1 to 5 Likert scale. Scores are calculated by summing the responses to each item for a given scale.

AWARENESS

RATING OPTIONS
1=None of the time; **2**=A little of the time; **3**=Some of the time;
4=A lot of the time; **5**=All of the time

1. When I want to focus, it's easy for me. _____
2. In general, I'm able to focus when I'm reading. _____

3. I can notice my thoughts as soon as I have them. _____

4. When some of my thoughts lead to other thoughts, I realize it while it is happening. _____

CONNECTION

RATING OPTIONS (ITEMS 1–3):
1=None of the time; **2**=A little of the time; **3**=Some of the time; **4**=A lot of the time; **5**=All of the time

1. I like all of the people that I see from day to day. _____
2. I actively take time to appreciate things about the people I see from day to day. _____
3. I believe that most people are doing the best they can. _____

RATING OPTIONS (ITEMS 4–6):
1=Not at all; **2**=A little bit; **3**=Somewhat; **4**=A lot; **5**=To the highest degree

4. I want all people to be happy, including people I don't like. _____
5. I care about the problems of people all over the world. _____
6. When I make decisions involving other people, I consider their best interests. _____

INSIGHT

RATING OPTIONS:
1=None of the time; **2**=A little of the time; **3**=Some of the time; **4**=Most of the time; **5**=All of the time

1. When I am interacting with someone, I reflect on how my feelings are causing me to treat them a certain way. _____
2. When I have a thought, I reflect on whether that thought is making me feel better or worse. _____
3. I can change how I feel about a situation by changing my thoughts about that situation. _____

PURPOSE

RATING OPTIONS:
1=Not at all; **2**=A little bit; **3**=Somewhat; **4**=A lot; **5**=To the highest degree

1. I have general life goals that make my daily activities worth doing. _____
2. I know what's really important in my life. _____
3. I have a life purpose that guides my day-to-day choices. _____
4. I know what kind of life I want to lead. _____

Transforming Everything into Practice

Getting some data on the four dimensions of flourishing is all well and good, but it won't do us much good if we never put the skills into practice. Imagine having a grand theory on tying your shoelaces or a perfect scientific framework for riding a bike—they would be pointless without practice. The power of understanding the four skills and what the data say about your current state is that it can help you see where the real opportunities are, the way a good physical shows you where some exercise or a change in diet might do the most good. At some point, we need to put down the book and hop on the treadmill. We need to practice.

The first question most people ask after getting their scores on the Healthy Minds Index is "How can I improve?" The simple answer is that there are many ways to learn and practice these skills. If you take the time to survey the world's wisdom traditions, you'll find an abundance of methods and techniques, from solitary meditation practices to interpersonal dialogue and discussion. There are movement-based practices like yoga and tai chi, and artistic traditions like calligraphy. Humans have invented seemingly endless forms of practice over the centuries.

Pretty much anything we do in life can be used as a practice to cultivate inner flourishing. In mapping the terrain of practice, we learned how Zen monks use sweeping and cleaning in the monastery to train attention and cultivate mindfulness and how some of the world's most well-known athletes include similar practices in their training. What transforms mundane activities into practices for flourishing isn't the activities themselves but rather the inner process that accompanies them. Simply sweeping a monastery won't make you happy or content, but if you go about your work with the motivation to be of benefit to others and a clear intention to be present and aware as you sweep, it has the potential to be deeply transformative and beneficial. The same is true of everything we do in life. With the right attitude, anything can be transformed into practice.

Hopefully, this clarifies what practice is all about. We often hear things like "Running is my meditation" or "Being in nature is my practice." Are these activities really flourishing practices? Well . . . maybe. There's no question that both physical exercise and being in nature support our ability to flourish, but are they practices in the same way as journaling and meditation? Again, the answer lies in the inner experience that accompanies the activity. Just having a calm, clear mind while you go for your morning jog doesn't magically transform it into meditation. What will make it a practice that supports your ability to flourish is a clear intention to train your mind while you are working out. While you go through the repetitive motions of jogging, for example, you could consciously choose to strengthen awareness by focusing on the sensations in your body, or you could cultivate appreciation by noticing positive things about the people and world around you. You could even generate insight by exploring all the beliefs and expectations you have about your body, or purpose by reflecting on your commitment to physical health as part of a larger sense of purpose in your life. Any one of these strategies or all of them in combination will transform your exercise routine into a meditation, but simply doing your usual routine without giving any thought to training your mind will not, no matter how calm and serene your mind may be when you do it.

Formal and Informal Practice

Distinguishing between formal and informal practice is also important. Formal practice does not necessarily mean sitting still in a quiet space. Rather, formal practice occurs when you set aside time with the specific intention to practice. This could be a twenty-minute meditation right after you wake up, but it could also be a period when you sit down to journal or do yoga after work. It could even be some mindful housework. As long as you have a clear intention to spend a period of time doing some activity as part of your practice, it becomes part of your formal practice. In other words, sitting perfectly still is not the only way to do a formal practice. There are many forms of active practice you can do while you are on the go and engaged in other activities.

Informal practice is what happens during the rest of your day, in all the moments when you spontaneously apply your training to daily life. If you're working on the skill of connection, for example, you might do a short gratitude reflection before you go to bed each night—that's the formal part—but the next day, when you run into a coworker and spontaneously make a point of letting them know you appreciate their support, that's an informal expression of your practice. Or, say you are working on insight. You might set aside five minutes over your lunch break to reflect on how you respond to stressful situations. That would be a formal practice. When you get home that night and find yourself in a stressful conversation with a family member, you might suddenly remember your reflection and spontaneously apply your insight in the moment to see your reaction more clearly—that would be a moment of informal practice.

The bottom line is that there are many ways to learn and practice the skills that help us flourish and even more ways to apply those skills in our lives. Meditation is perhaps the most well-known and widely studied way to practice, but it isn't the only way. The best practice, we often say, is the one you actually do. To give you the opportunity to experiment and explore, we've included a range of practices in the chapters that follow that you can try for yourself. We've also included sample practices for each of the four skills, including "The

Healthy Minds Meditation" that combines all four, in the appendix. So give them a try and see what works best for you. Our research shows that it only takes a few minutes a day—about 4.5 minutes—to derive real benefits, from relieving stress and anxiety to improving attention, social connections, and overall well-being. You can train your mind in just minutes a day.

Part Two

The Four Skills of Flourishing

Chapter 5

Awareness: The First Skill of Flourishing

This moment is all there is.

—Rumi

A year before moving to Madison to begin his doctoral work, Cort found himself lying in one of Richie's state-of-the-art fMRI brain scanners. He had signed up with a small group of experienced meditators to take part in a study of the brain's pain network (the regions known to be activated by physical pain). Richie and his colleague Antoine Lutz were asking a simple but important question: Do advanced meditators respond to pain like other people? Little did Cort know that to answer this question, he would need to lie for hours in the freezing-cold brain scanner, trying to meditate as Richie and his team of researchers found creative ways to inflict pain on him while observing his brain.

Lying in a scanner is surreal. Richie and Antoine had Cort lie on a hard platform that sticks out from the fMRI scanner, which looks like a giant plastic donut. Cort's head was positioned between foam pads so it couldn't move. With goggles plastered to his face and a small metal plate (a thermode) strapped to his wrist, he was pushed on the platform into the scanner, where he was told to stay perfectly still. The scanner clicked and whirred, then beeped at random intervals—not a relaxing environment—and then Cort was told to meditate.

The procedure was pretty straightforward. Cort would hear a sound at regular intervals, and seconds afterward, water would flow into the thermode. The temperature of the water was precisely calibrated. Sometimes, it was lukewarm, but half the time it was scalding hot—so hot that it would elicit an intense burning sensation a person could barely tolerate. Cort and 13 other meditators, as well as a control group of nonmeditators, had to endure 32 repetitions of this painful exercise while instructed to lie completely still and rest in a state of alert presence.

Many people would have yelped and ripped the thermode off, holding back expletives and wondering why on earth they'd signed up in the first place. But that's not what happened with Cort. As soon as he laid down, his meditation training kicked in. His practice had trained him to step back and observe the dynamic flow of inner experience with warm curiosity, so that's exactly what he did.

And the data were stunning. When Richie and Antoine analyzed the results, it confirmed their hypothesis that advanced meditators respond to pain differently. Unlike the nonmeditators, the response in the meditators' brains signaled far more emotional balance and inner calm. But the scientists also noticed something else. In nonmeditators, the brain's pain matrix wasn't active only during the painful stimulus but also *before* the pain even happened, and it stayed active long *after* the hot water was piped out of the thermode. It took time for the pain matrix to return to its baseline level. In other words, the nonmeditators were dealing with pain before and after the actual physical experience occurred. There seemed to be periods of anticipation and recovery in which the brain acted as if pain was still present when it was not.

Meanwhile, the experienced meditators had a completely different pattern of brain activity. In the period between the beeping sound and the arrival of the scalding-hot water—the same period when the nonmeditators anticipated what was about to happen—the meditators appeared to be in a calm, restful state. Their pain matrix did not grow active in the moments leading up to the pain, and once the pain ended, their pain matrix immediately returned to its normal activation level during the recovery period.

Richie and his team had discovered a stark contrast between the meditators and nonmeditators during the anticipation and recovery periods. The next question was whether there was a difference between them when the pain was actually present. Perhaps the meditators suppressed the experience of pain completely or at least dialed down the full impact of the scalding water. That's not what the data revealed. Not only was the pain matrix active in the meditators, but it was also *more* active than it was in the nonmeditators. Meditators were not screening out the pain. They seemed to be experiencing the pain more intensely, particularly in the brain's sensory regions linked to heat-related physical sensations.

At first glance, this seems counterintuitive. Why would it be a good thing to train your mind to experience pain more intensely? Well, it turns out that these discoveries about the pain matrix were only half the story. The scientists were examining not only brain activity in this study but also the participants' inner experience. After each trial, participants were asked to rate the intensity of the pain and indicate how unpleasant it was. The data showed that both groups rated the intensity about the same, while the meditators reported the pain as significantly less unpleasant. The meditators seemed to experience *pain without suffering*.

When Cort and the other meditators were lying in the scanner, they practiced meditation. Instead of ruminating on the pain, they focused on what was happening in the present moment. Cort himself didn't get stuck in anxious thoughts or anticipate when the pain would come and what it would be like. When the machine beeped, signaling that the hot water was about to arrive, he kept his awareness on his body in the present moment. He felt the movement of his breath. He noticed when his body started to tense up and brace itself for the pain, and as the thermode on his wrist grew hotter and hotter, he didn't try to distract himself or resist. He directed his attention straight to the pain, treating it like a fascinating new object in his awareness. He felt the flow of sensation as the pain rose and fell, noting all the physical, mental, and emotional reactions he was feeling while letting them pass by. When the hot water flowed out, he noticed the visceral sense of relaxation and relief in his body, again observing the dynamic flow of feelings and sensations in response to the pain's end.

If you had spoken with one of the nonmeditators, you would have heard a very different report. They complained. The experience was awful, and they could not let it go. Most were caught up in their judgments and reactions to what was happening. During the test, they wondered what would happen next and cursed the scientists for torturing them (or cursed themselves for signing up for such a stupid experiment). Unlike the meditators, they were probably oblivious to the rich array of details in the present moment, both the inner experience of bodily sensations and the whizzing, humming, and chirping of the fMRI scanner outside them.

The Power of Awareness

Our discovery with advanced meditators highlights a paradox of the human mind: challenging situations, even physical pain and emotional turmoil, are much less challenging when we are present and aware. Take a stressful situation like finding out you have to give a big presentation. Normally, you would do exactly what the nonmeditators did in the scanner. You might worry about the situation before it happens, wondering how it will go, what you'll say, how you'll feel, and how others will react. It's like you're doing a mental and emotional rehearsal, sometimes long before the event occurs. And it's the same thing all over again after the presentation. You might replay the memory over and over again while lying in bed that night. If you question whether it went well, you'll be stuck in a toxic swirl of thoughts and feelings.

Awareness gives you a different set of options. Instead of being hijacked by your reactions before, during, and after an event, you can slowly build the skill of noticing them as they come . . . and then go. When the email arrives with news about the big presentation, you can pause for a few mindful breaths to settle your nervous system. You can train yourself to respond with awareness instead of blindly reacting out of habit. You can set the worry aside and focus on the moment at hand. This same skill can help in countless daily life situations, from moments at work to time with family and friends and even in mundane moments when you're checking things off your daily to-do list.

Awareness is the first cornerstone of our ability to flourish.

What Is Awareness?

The human mind is complicated, filled with constantly changing mental states and psychological processes, both conscious and unconscious. Yet amid all this complexity, the mind has one ever-present quality: the knowing quality of consciousness itself. In our waking life, we all have a subjective knowing quality in our experience. If someone were to tap you on the shoulder and ask you what is happening, you could tell them. This knowing is awareness.

Simply having awareness is not enough for flourishing, however. We always have awareness, so clearly there is more to the picture. Our scientific research has confirmed that one of the key components of flourishing is *being in touch with awareness*. To use a crude analogy, having a priceless diamond in your pocket won't help you very much if you don't realize you have it or forget about it. You need to recognize what you have to truly benefit from it.

You've likely experienced moments of recognizing awareness. While reading this book, for example, there have probably been moments when your eyes have been scanning the page and taking in the visual shape of the letters, but your mind was elsewhere. You might even "read" an entire page without realizing you've lost touch with what the words are communicating. At some point, you will suddenly "wake up" to the fact that you've been distracted. This very recognition gives you the capacity to bring your mind back to what you are doing.

If you pay attention to that moment of wakeful awareness, you'll notice a heightened sense of presence. The words on the page might seem a little clearer and brighter. You might notice sounds and other sensory experiences, perhaps even sensations in your body or the quality of your mental state, that you didn't notice a moment earlier. In short, a moment of reconnecting with awareness is a rich inner experience compared with being distracted or losing yourself in what you are doing. There is a clear, palpable sense of being fully in the here and now.

Being in the here and now with our full presence is the key. In our research, we define awareness as "a heightened and flexible attentiveness" to what is happening in the moment, including what we see, hear, and feel, as well as the thoughts, emotions, memories, and impulses of our inner experience. "Heightened attentiveness" points to the wakeful quality of seeing the different aspects of our experience clearly. "Flexible attentiveness" points to the fact that we are in the driver's seat of our attention when we are in touch with awareness. Imagine walking outside on a beautiful summer day. You can feel the warmth of the sun and hear the birdsong. You pause to take it all in. That's awareness. But awareness is also there when you find yourself getting stressed out. Maybe you grow irritable or anxious over a thought, but instead of unconsciously allowing that thought to take you on a roller-coaster ride, you notice your reaction and take a breath before you react. That, too, is awareness.

PRACTICE

A Taste of Awareness

To get a taste for yourself, give this brief awareness practice a try:

Take a moment to look around you. Take in the rich world of shapes and colors. Notice some of the small details you usually don't pay attention to.

Next, gently close your eyes or leave them slightly open in a relaxed gaze. Take a few slow, deep breaths. As you breathe, bring awareness to the feeling of the air moving in and out of your body.

Now, notice the sounds in your environment or the silence if you're in a quiet space. Bring your full attention to whatever you hear at this moment.

You can end the practice by giving yourself a few moments to relax and rest. There's no need to concentrate or apply mental effort. Simply be present and take in the beauty of this moment.

Awareness Is a Skill

Until the last few decades, little scientific evidence linked awareness to our ability to flourish, and even less showed that awareness can be trained and strengthened. In fact, most scientific models of well-being and mental health don't even mention awareness. All that changed in the early 2000s with the explosion of research on mindfulness and other forms of meditation.

At the Center for Healthy Minds, we published some of the very first research in this area with our study of "Olympian" meditators. These advanced practitioners could seemingly trigger states of focused attention at will, with the most experienced practitioners able to sustain levels of heightened awareness almost effortlessly. Their mastery of awareness got all the attention, but what we found with the control group was also important. People with zero experience in meditation, once trained in awareness meditation practice, were able to activate the same brain networks linked to attention and awareness that the experts activated, just not to the same degree. This was the first hint that everyone, even a complete novice, can learn to cultivate awareness in a short period of time.

In today's world, many of us feel distracted and scattered much of the time. But for every moment of distraction, you likely have many more moments of awareness. We are all born with this innate quality. Brief moments of awareness happen frequently in daily life. When you don't eat breakfast and notice that you're feeling grumpy later in the day, that's a moment of awareness. When you're with a close friend and feel completely present, that's awareness, too, and when you're folding laundry or doing the dishes, you experience countless flashes of awareness. These moments are so common we don't even notice them.

The skill of awareness is training ourselves to recognize and then nurture these moments of wakeful presence. Every time you recognize a moment of awareness, related brain networks are activated, and you strengthen your ability to be a more attentive listener, focus on your work, or better manage your emotional reactions and habitual impulses. All of these experiences enhance flourishing.

When you connect with awareness, what you will likely find is that the full range of human experience feels better. You can savor peak experiences when you're fully present. You'll be more resilient in the face of setbacks, whether a minor irritation or a major challenge. Even boring routines and chores can become fulfilling and meaningful when you use them as opportunities to train the skill of awareness. Simply put, awareness is your normal, everyday life . . . but better.

Both of us have been practicing the skill of awareness for decades, and over the years, we've found countless ways to bring more awareness into our everyday lives. Cort used to be restless and easily bored, but now he savors the moments when there's nothing to do except wait. In moments when most people pull out their phones or find some other way to kill some time, he takes the opportunity to practice being present and aware, transforming what might otherwise be a meaningless period of distraction into something more nourishing and energizing. Richie does the same with mundane household chores. Instead of doing the dishes mindlessly, he turns the activity into an awareness practice by consciously paying attention to all the sounds and the feeling of the water on his hands. This might not sound exciting if you haven't learned these skills yourself, but if you take the time to cultivate awareness, mundane moments can become gateways to inner calm and joy.

There are two main benefits of awareness, both of which support our ability to flourish. First, it feels good to be aware. When we're scattered and distracted, we're more stressed. As we saw in chapter 3, distraction causes us to be on autopilot, driven by habits and impulses, which is an exhausting way to live. The closest we'll get to feeling content will be to lose ourselves in distraction, but succumbing to the pull of distraction is like drinking salt water, which leaves us worse off than where we started. Being aware, on the other hand, is a deeply nourishing experience. The second main benefit of awareness is that it helps us manage our thoughts, emotions, and impulses. In scientific terms, we call this "top-down self-regulation," one of the gifts of flourishing. We can consciously regulate our mental and emotional states instead of being controlled by them. When we get triggered or feel an unhealthy impulse, we have the ability to notice what's happening in our mind and body before getting swept away by the current. Awareness is a critical ingredient of willpower and self-mastery.

Your Brain on Awareness

Awareness practices strengthen two brain networks that are critical for self-regulation: the central executive network and the salience network, which we mentioned in chapter 2.

The executive network is a group of brain regions located primarily in the prefrontal cortex, the part of your brain just behind your forehead. This network is involved in decision-making, problem-solving, attentional focus, and goal-directed behavior. It also plays a central role in various forms of self-regulation. If you have some important work to do, this is the network that will help you stay focused on the task and deal with any challenges along the way. This network is also responsible for helping you break a bad habit or build a healthy one, and it can help you manage a strong emotional reaction when you get frustrated or anxious.

The regions that comprise the salience network are buried deeper in the brain and play a different role. The salience network grows active when you notice something important or need to monitor a situation to respond appropriately. If you're in a tense conversation and suddenly notice an impulse to say something unkind, that moment of noticing activates the salience network. If you're cooking dinner and need to keep an eye on what you're cooking, your ability to monitor the situation and make sure nothing gets burned also activates this network.

This ability to watch, observe, and notice sets the stage for self-regulation. For example, let's say you feel your phone vibrating in your pocket. Usually, you'll pull it out without thinking, but if you're trying to be more intentional about checking your messages, you might notice the impulse before taking action. That's the salience network. That moment of noticing the impulse will give you a new set of options. You can consciously regulate your response, which reflects the activation of the executive network. You might choose to ignore the impulse, or you could check your message mindfully and intentionally instead of out of blind habit. The executive and salience networks thus work together.

The salience network can also "recruit" other brain regions and networks, including the executive network, to mobilize the right response. In some cases, it might activate the amygdala, a brain region linked to emotions and feelings, to trigger an emotional response. In other cases, it might mobilize the executive network to manage a toxic train of thoughts or help you control a strong emotional reaction. In both cases, the salience network functions as a traffic cop that monitors things and ensures the brain responds appropriately.

When you practice awareness, you are learning to balance the salience and executive networks. Strengthening these networks is a lot like strengthening your immune system. It will make your mind strong and resilient, not only in the few minutes you spend doing an awareness practice but also in virtually every other situation. Whether you're with family or friends, crossing things off your to-do list, or just going about your day, keeping these networks strong and healthy will help you stay calm and balanced, even in stressful situations.

Mindfulness, Meta-Awareness, and Experiential Fusion

The terms *mindfulness* and *awareness* are often used interchangeably, but they have different meanings. A classic definition of mindfulness is "the act of remaining aware of a given object without forgetting it." If you are meditating and aware of your breath, you are mindful; when you get distracted and forget, mindfulness is lost. If you are meditating on compassion by keeping your attention on someone and nurturing a feeling of warmth and care, you are mindful. But when you forget and your mind wanders, you are no longer mindful. In essence, mindfulness is the process of remembering to be aware.

In a scientific paper we published in 2015, we referred to the movement from distraction to awareness as a shift from "experiential fusion" to "meta-awareness." Experiential fusion is just a fancy scientific term for the experience of being lost or absorbed. This includes moments of garden-variety distraction and periods when you're just going through the motions with only a dim awareness of what you are doing. Have you ever driven somewhere and suddenly realized you were zoned out and distracted? Or maybe you're in the middle of a conversation and find yourself thinking about something else, with no idea what the other person just said. In such moments, you might be so caught up in your thoughts or so lost in what you're doing that it feels like you're "fused" with what you are experiencing. If you're thinking about something, you *are* the thoughts. If you're angry, you *are* the anger. There's no space between you and the experience you're having. That's experiential fusion.

Meta-awareness is the opposite of experiential fusion. With

meta-awareness, you're aware of what is happening in your mind. If you are thinking, you are not lost in thoughts when you know you are thinking. If you are doing something with meta-awareness, there is a sense of presence: you are aware of what you are doing while doing it. And if you have an emotional response, whether a pleasant emotion like joy or a challenging one like fear, you know the emotion is happening. It doesn't hijack your inner experience.

You can explore the difference between experiential fusion and meta-awareness in any situation, including right now while you're reading. Whether you're absorbed in the process of reading or distracted, the fact that you're reading about meta-awareness might trigger an experience in this very moment. Notice if you can read with a heightened sense of presence. You are still reading, as you have a million other times in your life, but with a fuller experience of awareness.

Can you sense the difference? In a way, nothing is different. It's just you reading. Nothing too extraordinary. On the other hand, the presence of meta-awareness will shift your experience in a few important ways. First, you will likely have a richer, deeper experience of what you are doing. You might notice subtle details about the experience of reading that you normally miss, like the colors and textures you see, the voice in your head, or the images that occur as you process the words on the page. Connecting to awareness in this way will give you the ability to manage your attention. If you wanted, you could shift your attention to the sounds in your environment, the thoughts in your mind, or some other experience. This shift into awareness can be described as a moment of mindfulness or an experience of meta-awareness. However you describe it, it is a deeply nourishing and transformative experience.

What About Flow?

If we were having a public discussion about these topics, at this point someone in the room would raise their hand and ask about the experience of flow. Their questions would likely run along these lines: Isn't being completely absorbed in an activity the same as flow? Is flow a good form of distraction? Is it the same thing as awareness? And isn't flow a good thing? Don't we want more flow in our lives?

The simple answer is that there are many kinds of flow, and some of them are better than others when it comes to awareness. Flow is a concept that was studied by an important psychologist named Mihaly Csikszentmihalyi, who described it as the experience of being so completely focused on a particular activity and absorbed in the moment that time seems to slow down and the self drops away. At the far end of the spectrum are virtuoso performances, like a champion athlete playing the perfect game or a musician playing a difficult piece to perfection. They use their skills and abilities to the maximum, and the perfect move spontaneously happens at just the right moment. Outside of these peak experiences are the more ordinary states of flow. You might be working on something with such laser focus that you lose track of time. This can happen when you're absorbed in your work, in a moment of deep connection with friends or a romantic partner, or when enjoying the serenity of the natural world.

Experiences of flow can happen with or without meta-awareness. In both cases, the experience of self and time drop away. When flow occurs with meta-awareness, you will also experience a strong, visceral sense of presence. The world of the senses will open up. It might feel like what you see is more vivid and what you hear is clearer and crisper. You may feel a sense of joy or deep ease and contentment, as though all is right with the world. However, when meta-awareness is not present, you may get that same sense of timelessness and lose your sense of self, but it will feel as though awareness has grown dim, not brighter. You will likely feel "lost" in the activity, almost like you've fallen asleep, only to "wake up" once the flow state ends.

Cultivating awareness will help you experience more flow in your life with the benefit of meta-awareness. You will get in the zone when you want or need to without losing your ability to manage your mental and emotional states. This is the path to self-mastery, and it takes just a few minutes of practice each day.

Building an Awareness Practice

If we look to Jon Kabat-Zinn's excellent definition of mindfulness—"the awareness that emerges through paying attention on purpose, in the present moment, and nonjudgmentally to the unfolding of experience moment by moment"—we find all the ingredients we need to build a strong awareness practice. Jon Kabat-Zinn, of course, is a well-known author and teacher of mindfulness and the founder of the Mindfulness-Based Stress Reduction Clinic and the Center for Mindfulness in Medicine, Health Care, and Society at UMass Memorial Health.

Kabat-Zinn's elegant definition captures the three key elements of cultivating awareness *as a skill*: intention, presence, and attention. Let's look at these one by one.

Intention is paying attention "on purpose," as Kabat-Zinn put it. Moments of mindful awareness happen naturally all the time, but practicing awareness as a skill takes intention. You notice moments of awareness when they happen on purpose; you consciously nurture them. You also notice moments of distraction and absorption when the light of awareness dims. This quality of intention is one important key to discerning whether something is or is not an awareness practice. We've commented that people often say things like "Jogging is my meditation" or "Being in nature is my meditation." Are these activities really meditation? It depends. Jogging and being in nature can indeed be used as ways to sharpen the skill of awareness, but as we mentioned earlier, jogging is not a meditative practice simply because your mind is more peaceful and calm when you do it. It takes intention. If you attend to what is happening in the moments while you jog, consciously and intentionally, then it becomes an awareness practice. The key distinction is the presence or absence of intention.

The second element of an awareness practice is presence, which simply means you are oriented to what is happening in the here and now. The here and now might be the process of breathing if you are meditating or listening closely to what a friend is saying if you are in a social setting. It could even mean being present to your own thoughts and feelings if you are learning to be self-aware of your reactions and impulses in the here and now. In scientific terms, you might say that this element of awareness practice points to meta-awareness. If meta-awareness is active, you are present. If it isn't, you are not.

The third element of an awareness practice is attention. In all forms of awareness practice, from mindfulness meditation to a physical activity like yoga, you are doing something very specific with your attentional focus. To a large degree, the skill of awareness involves training attention. You might have a broad, panoramic field of attention or a laser-like focus. Your practice might have you concentrating with great effort or relaxing into effortless presence. Whatever else might be involved, you will be doing something specific with your attention.

There are a range of ways you can practice the skill of attention. There are "object-oriented" practices where you focus on your breath, a sound, a visual object, or even a particular thought, feeling, or emotion. In some practices, you pick one object and stay with it. In others, you bring your attention to everything that naturally enters your field of awareness, a practice sometimes referred to as "open monitoring" or "choiceless awareness." On the other end of the spectrum are "subject-oriented" practices where you attend to awareness itself rather than the objects of awareness. Unlike "object-oriented" practices, which often have a more laser-like focus, the mind becomes very open and expansive. "Open awareness" and "open presence" meditations are common examples of subject-oriented practices.

All of these variations sharpen the skill of awareness and involve the three elements of intention, presence, and attention. Let's see how these elements play out in open awareness meditation, the core form of awareness practice.

PRACTICE

Open Awareness Meditation

There are many ways to practice the skill of awareness, from using sensory experiences like the breath or bodily sensations as a support to the cultivation of self-awareness by observing thoughts. However, if we had to pick one practice, it would be open awareness meditation. Open awareness is all about the lost art of being. It's subtle and challenging, and it helps us see that our true value and worth as human beings is not what we do and accomplish but who we are.

The ability to let go and simply be aware is one of the most critical elements on the path to flourishing. Yet the fast pace of life in the twenty-first century gives us precious little time to rest and recharge. Our lives can be so consumed by "doing" that simply "being" can feel like a foreign concept. Open awareness meditation helps us relearn how to be in awareness itself. In this brief practice, you will explore the shift from doing to being by resting in a state of effortless, open presence.

To begin, sit in a comfortable posture and ground yourself with a few slow, calming breaths. You can keep your eyes open or closed, whichever feels more natural.

Set an uplifting motivation for your practice by envisioning how cultivating awareness might enrich your life and ripple out to benefit others.

When you feel ready, set an intention to be fully present for this short exercise. You can start by bringing awareness to your breath. You don't need to focus or concentrate; simply note that you are breathing and feel the movement of your breath in and out of your body.

As you breathe, allow yourself to shift from a state of doing to being, to a state of effortless presence. There is nothing particular to "do" here. Give yourself time and space simply to exist. Just breathe, with a very light touch of awareness.

Next, you can let go of your focus on your breath and rest naturally in awareness for a few moments. You don't need to do anything or change anything. Simply exist, as you are, in this moment.

Let go of any impulse to focus or concentrate your attention. Instead, widen the aperture of your attention and rest in a state of open, effortless awareness. If this feels unfamiliar or you're not sure what to "do," just sit here and enjoy the present moment.

When your mind wanders, notice it has without judgment, and then continue to rest in awareness, without applying any mental effort or trying to change or improve what's happening in the present moment.

> To conclude your practice, open your eyes if they are closed, look around, and take in the beauty of this moment.
>
> As you continue reading or transition into whatever comes next in your day, pause from time to time and rest in open, effortless awareness. You can scatter many short moments of awareness throughout your day.

Many Ways to Cultivate Awareness

While open awareness practice will, without a doubt, improve your skill with awareness, almost any activity can become a vehicle for strengthening the skill. The great philosophers of the Western world, from Marcus Aurelius to Henry David Thoreau, used self-reflection and time in nature to cultivate awareness. Christian mystics have found awareness through prayer. And in various traditions, physical movement is offered as a gateway to awareness. Consider the meditative dance of Islam's Sufi tradition, the flowing movements in tai chi, the precise postures of hatha yoga, and the martial arts of East Asia. You can also find awareness-based artistic traditions, where the creative process is linked to intentionally cultivating awareness. In Japan, for example, many of the masterpieces of calligraphy, poetry, painting, and even flower arrangement were created by meditation masters. Today, there are mindfulness classes for just about everything, from parenting to cooking and knitting. If you have a hobby or a passion, there's probably a mindfulness class to help you do it with more awareness.

You can also bring the elements of awareness—intention, attention, and presence—to your social interactions. The decision to use your interactions as an opportunity to practice this skill is itself a form of intention. You might pick a specific situation for your practice, like sitting around the dinner table or a particular time with friends. When you find yourself in the situation, you could remind yourself of your intention and then consciously choose to be present and aware of the people you're with.

As you practice in social situations, you might notice that social awareness requires a different form of attention from other practices. Your field of awareness might be more relaxed and expansive when you're interacting with people than when you're practicing mindful breathing and your attentional focus is narrow. You might focus most of your attention on the people you are with, taking in what they are saying, their facial expressions and gestures, as well as the broader context and environment. You might also have a light awareness of your internal mental and physical states as you interact with others. You might notice your impulse to jump in and comment when someone is sharing a story or notice a flash of tension when someone says something that irritates you.

We like to practice awareness when out for a walk or a bike ride. On a walk, you can use the world of the senses—what you see, hear, and smell—as the object of awareness. On a bike ride, Richie enjoys being aware of all his senses both for the pleasure of the ride and for safety. When doing the dishes, the laundry, or another chore, you can use the tactile sensation of touch or the sounds of the activity as your practice. When exercising, you can use the feelings in your body or the movement of your breath. In short, lean in and explore the experience of whatever you are doing and whoever you are with. With this approach, everything becomes an opportunity to practice.

Rewiring the Brain with Awareness

After just a few weeks of practicing open awareness or practicing awareness while folding the laundry or going for a walk, you will begin to feel calmer and more settled. You will be on the road to flourishing. But there's even more exciting news: your brain will actually change along with the changes you're feeling. In one study at the Center for Healthy Minds, we recruited a group of 40 experienced meditators to measure how the brain changes with awareness practice. They were not the "Olympian" meditators of our early research; they were everyday people with jobs and families who had maintained a regular meditation practice for at least five years. We also recruited a control group of 124 nonmeditators. In each of these groups, we examined patterns of brain activity during what scientists call the "resting state," which refers to a period when someone is not engaged in a particular activity or task. To measure their "resting state" brain activity, we put all our subjects in an MRI scanner and instructed them to lie still for a series of scans.

We discovered that the meditators' brains behaved very differently from those of the nonmeditators. The meditators had stronger connections between the brain regions responsible for self-regulation and other areas linked to mind-wandering and rumination. This is exactly what we had hoped to find. It supported the idea that cultivating awareness strengthens our ability to notice and regulate mental and emotional states, including distracted mind-wandering. We also found weaker connections within the brain regions linked to distraction (the "default-mode" network). And we were pleasantly surprised to find these differences when the subjects were in the scanner doing nothing, not when they were meditating. The takeaway? Awareness practice is not only beneficial when we are actually practicing awareness but has a "spillover" effect that changes the way our brains function as we go about our day.

In another study, we recruited roughly 150 subjects and put them into three groups. One was a control group that did no awareness practice during the study. A second group was an "active" control. They participated in a Health Enhancement Program that included a range of practical instructions to boost well-being but no instructions related to awareness. The third group—the main experimental focus of our study—participated in an eight-week training in awareness practice, the well-known Mindfulness-Based Stress Reduction (MBSR) Program created by Jon Kabat-Zinn.

After the eight-week training, our previous results from other studies were further confirmed. We found stronger connectivity between a key brain region responsible for self-regulation (the dorsolateral prefrontal cortex) and a central node of the brain's default-mode network (the network that underlies distraction and mind-wandering)—and we also found that this connection was linked to how much people practiced awareness. The more time someone spends cultivating awareness, the stronger these connections will be. However, the more sobering finding was that the improvements from awareness practice don't necessarily last. These connections had faded when we measured them a few months after the training. Taken altogether, these promising findings confirm that even complete beginners can experience rapid improvements, although it will take continued practice to sustain the benefits.

The World Needs Awareness

We are living in an age of anxiety and distraction. As we've noted, our minds are facing unprecedented levels of stress: the endless scroll of our social media feeds, the barrage of information from the 24/7 news cycle, and the seemingly endless stream of global crises and upheaval. All this stress takes a toll on our relationships, physical health, and emotional well-being. We all feel the toxic effects.

Awareness gives us our power back. It gives us confidence and the autonomy to choose how we want to live. From Buddhist monks living in caves high on the Tibetan plateau to towering figures of modern psychology, from the Stoic philosophers of ancient Greece and Rome to the wandering Christian mystics and the Sufi poets of Islam, humans have long known that the mind possesses untapped potential to be present and aware and that when we take the time to nurture this potential, it can transform every aspect of our lives. Practicing the skill of awareness will make you a better listener with the people you care about and give you more focus at work. It will help you savor your peak moments and navigate life's pains and sorrows. In between the highs and lows, cultivating awareness will put you in touch with a deep reservoir of inner calm that you can carry through all the mundane moments of your daily routine. Awareness is the first of the greatest inner resources we possess to flourish. Making full use of it is no longer a luxury. It is a necessity.

Chapter 6

Connection: The Second Skill of Flourishing

My religion is kindness.

—The Dalai Lama

Richie stood next to the Dalai Lama at the end of a long corridor, watching patients being wheeled out of their rooms. His mind was filled with doubt. His Holiness was visiting the National Institutes of Health (NIH) for the first time, something Richie had been trying to make happen for years. His lab has been continuously funded by the NIH for forty-five years. For the first thirty years, it would not fund any of his meditation research; only in the last fifteen years has the NIH included meditation as a legitimate area for funding. By having the Dalai Lama speak at the NIH, Richie was hoping to catalyze their interest in contemplative science and the science of flourishing.

Once Francis Collins stepped in as the director of the NIH, the Dalai Lama's visit became possible. When Richie reached out to Francis, a towering figure in modern genetics (he was director of the Human Genome Project) and a deeply spiritual man, he responded positively—a controversial decision on his part. The NIH is the holiest of holy cathedrals in modern science. Inviting a spiritual figure like the Dalai Lama was anathema to many scientists. Nevertheless, Francis shared our views on the value of bringing science and spirituality into conversation, and we set out planning the visit.

Francis suggested we bring the Dalai Lama to some of the NIH's research facilities. "We've got some of the most high-tech research tools on the planet," he mused, "and the Dalai Lama loves engineering and hardware, from what I've heard. Why don't we take him to see some of the labs?"

Richie gave it some thought, remembering the many trips His Holiness had made to the UW–Madison lab and other universities and scientific labs. "That might be interesting, but he's already been to some of the world's best research centers. What if we do something completely different?"

We bounced some ideas back and forth, but nothing stuck. "What if we visit the hospital on the NIH campus?" Richie asked. "He loves meeting and interacting with people, especially if he can comfort those who are suffering. What do you think?"

A year later, in March 2014, we were all in the hospital corridor. Francis and Richie stood next to His Holiness. We were surrounded by an unlikely entourage of maroon-robed Buddhist monks and some of the leading scientists at the NIH, many of whom were the most influential in the world. A number of the patients the hospital staff wheeled out into the hallway were terminally ill. All were suffering. For the next sixty minutes, Francis, Richie, the scientists, and the NIH leaders witnessed a series of interactions we will never forget.

Helped along by an attendant, the Dalai Lama slowly shuffled down the hallway and met with the patients one by one. He didn't know any of these people, and they didn't know him. Some probably didn't know who he was or only vaguely recognized him. Yet, despite the lack of familiarity that would typically make a first interaction stiff and formal, the Dalai Lama greeted each person like a long-lost friend he hadn't seen in years. "Oh, so wonderful to see you!" he would exclaim, taking their hands in his and holding them warmly. "How are you feeling? Thank you for taking the time to greet an old man like me."

Such unbridled enthusiasm might seem fake or artificial with anyone else, but the Dalai Lama radiates authenticity. His words and demeanor are so genuine you cannot help but be deeply moved by his compassion. One by one, people blossomed in the warmth of his care and affection. They spoke. He listened. Occasionally, he asked questions about their condition, the treatment they were receiving, or their lives and families. It wasn't long before all the patients were beaming with smiles, crying, or both. There wasn't a dry eye in that entire hallway.

The Power of Connection

Richie's encounter in the hospital corridor at the NIH was hardly an everyday interaction, not only because it involved the Dalai Lama. What stood out was the healing power of deep human connection. Connection, even for a few moments, has a tremendous power to uplift and heal.

Richie and Cort have both seen the Dalai Lama meet and interact with people many times before and since his visit to the NIH. What was it about how he interacted with the patients that day that made it so impactful? Although it's hard to put a finger on it, we think it was the combination of the raw suffering of the people the Dalai Lama met and the unconditional love, care, and concern he spontaneously expressed in response. Just witnessing his genuine compassion was transformative.

His ability to connect did not just contribute to the patients' flourishing that day. It's also a significant part of the Dalai Lama's ability to flourish. If we all cultivated some of the compassion and kindness skills the Dalai Lama exhibited that day, we would be further along the path of flourishing. The Dalai Lama has spent thousands of hours nurturing qualities like kindness and compassion, both of which are foundational for the ability to connect. He has also trained himself to see the very best in others, to stay open to their suffering, and to provide care in whatever way he can. Like professional athletes who train themselves to respond in just the right way at just the right moment, what Richie witnessed that day was the result of a lifetime of steady practice.

What Is Connection?

In our research, we define connection as "an inner sense of care and kinship that leads to supportive interactions and caring relationships with others." Feelings of connection happen naturally and spontaneously when we experience positive social emotions like appreciation, kindness, and compassion, just as they evaporate in the heat of apathy, anger, and fear. Imagine yourself in any social situation to see how these inner states shape how connected you feel to others. Let's say you're at work, and a colleague gets promoted. You could respond in several ways. If you feel a burst of appreciation for their skills and rejoice in their good fortune, your appreciation will bring a feeling of connection, kinship, and care. But if you feel envious or focus on your colleague's negative qualities, that feeling of connection will be lost. Or let's say you're grabbing some coffee and notice that the barista is stressed out by the long line of customers. You might experience a moment of compassion, which will spark a feeling of connection to this complete stranger. But if you're too caught up in your busy day to notice, you'll feel apathy instead.

Although many social emotions can trigger feelings of connection, our research specifically focuses on appreciation, kindness, and compassion. Each of these emotions plays a unique role in fostering a sense of connection. We've chosen to track these three because they also play a unique role in supporting our ability to flourish. *Appreciation* occurs when we focus on something positive in another person, like noticing that a friend has a great sense of humor. *Kindness* is a movement toward happiness. When we smile at someone to brighten their day, for example, we naturally want them to be happy. That's kindness. *Compassion* comes from a space of warmhearted connection that is focused on relieving another's hardship and suffering. Compassion drives us toward care. For example, when a loved one loses their job, we make time to be with them.

Feelings of connection can manifest in many ways. In some situations, connection shows up as your ability to care for others. For example, it might mean that you sacrifice some of your time and energy to help someone in a time of need or that you put in the time to maintain an important relationship. At other times, connection manifests as your ability to be on the receiving end of someone else's care. You are willing to let that person in, to be vulnerable and open to their compassion. Connection might allow you to feel supported as you work through a difficult life transition, or it might allow you to know that someone has your back when you stand up for yourself at work. Connection can also simply be having people in your life you trust will be there for you in a time of need.

Caring relationships and interactions shape our mental health and emotional well-being like nothing else. Think about this in your own life. Can you recall a time when you felt deeply connected and supported by someone? Or how about a time when you stepped up in a relationship and were at your very best as a parent, partner, or friend? How did your sense of connection in these moments impact the rest of your life? If you're like most people, that feeling of strong social connection hugely boosts many areas of your life. Even reflecting on moments of connection gives us a boost.

In chapter 3, we considered some of the devastating consequences of feeling disconnected. What about times you've felt disconnected? Think back to a period when you felt lonely or isolated. How did that ripple out to the rest of your life? How did it affect the quality of your work and your ability to stay focused? Many of us become depressed or anxious when we don't feel connection in our lives, and it often colors everything we do. We get stressed out and overwhelmed more easily, doing our best work is hard, and we might find ourselves following our worst impulses and making unhealthy decisions.

The important thing to recognize here is that connection is all about our feelings. There is a crucial difference between our objective connections (how many people we see and interact with) and our feelings about these connections. In other words, *feeling connected* is an inner experience, and our inner experience can be very different from what's happening outside. If you're sitting by yourself and thinking about someone you care about with warm, caring thoughts, you'll probably feel deeply connected. But if you're struggling at work and feel unsupported even though you're surrounded by other people, you won't feel connected. The number of relationships and interactions we have with others matters, but how we feel about them matters more.

Scientists have studied the phenomenon of feeling alone in a crowd. It turns out that feeling lonely has only a modest link to objective social factors like how isolated you are, how many people you have in your social network, and how much support they give you. More important is how you feel about your relationships, particularly how supported you feel. If your life is filled with friends and family, but you don't feel supported, then all the interactions in the world won't add to your well-being. Decades of scientific research and thousands of years of accumulated wisdom from the world's wisdom traditions point to the importance of feeling connected as a core dimension of flourishing.

Our research mirrors this important distinction between the "objective" and "subjective" aspects of social connection. When we worked with schoolteachers during the Covid-19 pandemic, we discovered that strengthening their feelings of connection played an important role in helping them reduce overwhelming levels of stress, anxiety, and depression. We asked them to do one of our five connection-building activities each day for a month. They could choose to do a sitting meditation or one of the more active, "on the go" practices. They never had to do more than five minutes at a time unless they wanted to practice longer. We found that the time they spent cultivating connection made a substantial difference in their mental health and emotional well-being. When we measured the teachers a month later, their feelings of loneliness had decreased by 20 percent—even more heartening, these improvements were still there, with only a small decrease, when we measured them again three months later. (We will teach some of these practices in this chapter, and you will find others in the appendix.)

Increases in connection played an outsized role in reducing the anxiety, depression, and stress so many teachers and school employees were dealing with at the peak of the pandemic. In a second phase of analysis, our colleague Matt Hirshberg (the lead scientist on this study) found that decreases in loneliness accounted for a whopping 63 percent of the improvements we saw in stress, anxiety, and depression. This was a surprising discovery that showed no matter how lonely and isolated our circumstances might be, we can still cultivate a sense of connection, and doing so can have a powerful effect on our ability to weather life's storms.

Imagine what this might look like in your own life. Say you're experiencing an unexpected loss that leaves you feeling completely alone. Your circumstances might be out of your control, but your feelings are another matter. While you give yourself space to feel the sadness that accompanies the loss, you can also temper your grief with nourishing emotions like appreciation and gratitude. You might reflect on the warm memories or positive qualities of the person or thing you lost, bring other people and situations to mind that you also appreciate, or imagine future scenarios when you feel deeply connected.

This is exactly what happened with Cort's wife, Kasumi, who lost her sister to cancer a few years ago. Kasumi was very close to her sister and spent months caring for her during her illness in her home country of Japan. When her sister passed away after an agonizing year spent in hospitals, Kasumi was devastated. Her sister was only in her thirties when she died. Kasumi grieved her absence and all the life she didn't get to live, but amid the grief, Kasumi also recalled her sister's quirky ways and the laughs they'd shared. Her heart swelled with gratitude for the time they had together. This didn't make her sadness go away—nor did Kasumi want it to—but it did help her grieve the loss with a heart that felt full rather than empty.

PRACTICE

A Taste of Connection

True connection with others, even brief moments with strangers, and our ability to feel the connection are vital for our mental and physical health. We become more resilient in the face of challenges, more productive at work, and more energized with the things we care about. Feeling connected even supports our immune system. Simply put, feeling connected is one of the most important dimensions of flourishing.

To get a taste of the practice of connection, pause for a few minutes and follow these steps:

Start by bringing yourself fully into this moment. Take a few slow, deep breaths, center yourself, and when you're ready, begin the following reflection.

Think about people who have cared for you or supported you in your life. Who comes to mind? See if you can find one specific person and reflect on the different ways their presence has enriched your life. What do you most appreciate about this person?

Now, think about the ways you have helped or supported others. How do you express kindness and compassion? See if you can find at least one or two ways, small or large, that you have enriched someone else's life.

For the final step, imagine ways you could practice the skill of connection in the next day or two. It could be as simple as sending a nice message to someone. Use your imagination and envision yourself expressing care in some small way.

Connection Is a Skill

Connection practices can play a critical role in helping us make the leap from feeling isolated to finding meaningful human bonds, even in challenging circumstances. This was the case for Miguel, a software engineer who found himself struggling with a profound sense of disconnection when his company transitioned to fully remote work.

Though surrounded by digital faces all day, Miguel felt increasingly isolated. Video calls remained strictly technical, and the casual conversations that had once energized his workday—those spontaneous interactions in hallways and break rooms that naturally nurtured workplace relationships—had vanished. His productivity declined, and he began contemplating changing jobs. The screen that was meant to connect him to colleagues had become a barrier instead.

Miguel decided to try a different approach. He began practicing appreciation intentionally. Before each virtual meeting, he would take thirty seconds to reflect on something he genuinely valued about each colleague he was about to see—one person's creativity in solving problems, another's reliability in meeting deadlines, someone else's ability to explain complex concepts clearly.

When he felt the gravitational pull of isolation during his workday, he would express his appreciation in small ways—acknowledging specific contributions in meetings, sending brief notes of thanks, or simply beginning conversations with authentic interest in others' experiences. "May we all find meaning in our work today," he would sometimes think silently at the start of team calls, like a personal mantra. Linking his experience to appreciation immediately defused the emotional charge of his disconnection.

These simple practices changed how Miguel approached interactions, creating space for real connection even across digital divides. His colleagues began responding in kind, and the team culture gradually shifted toward greater openness and support. What had been a mechanical exchange of information slowly transformed into a community of individuals who felt seen and valued.

Many of us think that strengthening our sense of connection is simply a matter of spending more time with people, but it's a little more complicated than that. We can feel deeply connected to people across digital divides, and we can also feel completely alone on crowded video calls with people we've known for years. We can't always control the external circumstances of our work lives, but we can work on how we respond. In the decades we've spent learning and studying connection, we've heard from many people who say practicing this skill of connection and feeling connected has changed their lives.

Born to Connect

Practicing the skill of feeling connected is easier than you might think. It's a matter of noticing the moments of connection that happen spontaneously all the time and then nurturing them. If you know where to look, you will see these sparks of connection everywhere—small gestures of kindness, moments of cooperation, and experiences of gratitude. If you really pay attention, you'll quickly see that the impulse to connect is innate and automatic.

The challenge is that moments of connection are so common we rarely notice them. Instead, we notice the moments of disconnection. We notice these because they are *not* the norm. They stand out. If you commute to work or drive around town, for example, you will probably notice moments when people don't play by the rules. Someone cuts you off in traffic. Another person goes too fast or too slow. Someone else seems to be texting while driving. What you probably won't notice are the countless moments of seamless social harmony—tens or even hundreds of complete strangers all moving together, like a well-choreographed dance. The negative moments in a morning commute stand out because they are out of the ordinary. Social harmony is the norm.

Most of our lives proceed in this way. You might remember painful moments when a coworker didn't give you credit for some important work or when a friend or family member forgot an important event in your life. You will definitely remember times when someone did something really hurtful or unkind or when you were the one who hurt someone else. You probably won't think twice about the countless moments of connection you experience. There are many flashes of appreciation and care every single day, times when you spontaneously lend a helping hand, offer a kind word, or notice something nice about another person. Even in an everyday situation like getting groceries, there are fleeting experiences of kindness—but if you're scrolling through your phone, you'll miss them. You might miss the warm interactions of a family choosing a cereal or how one person spontaneously makes room for another trying to get through a busy aisle. These moments of subtle connection happen far more frequently than social discord and tension, but they usually go unnoticed.

We are social creatures by nature. From the time we are infants, we seek out warm, caring interactions and pull away from the aggressive or unfriendly ones. We recognize when others are hurt or suffering and feel the spontaneous movement to help. Our social drives are also mirrored in our biology. From the care network in our brains to chemicals like oxytocin that help us support others and feel supported, our entire nervous system has evolved to promote strong social ties. We are hardwired to connect.

Practicing the Skill of Connection

Recognizing moments of appreciation, kindness, and compassion will get you started on the path of practicing the skill of connection. But how do you take fleeting moments of connection and turn them into a steady practice? How do you strengthen positive connections with the people you care about and bring more kindness into your interactions and relationships? His Holiness the Dalai Lama famously gets up at 3 a.m. to practice, and compassion is one of his go-to meditations. There are two steps to practicing this skill and many different practices that incorporate one or both of these steps. Luckily, neither requires getting up at 3 a.m. or practicing for tens of thousands of hours.

The first step is to generate feelings like appreciation, kindness, and care with people and situations where these feelings come naturally. The second is to gradually widen your circle of connection to include more and more people until no one is left out. Eventually, you can train yourself to respond with warmth and care even in stressful situations, with people you don't know very well, or with people you find challenging. Compassion will become natural and automatic. It takes a lifetime to truly master this skill, as we see with the Dalai Lama, but we can still experience the benefits from small amounts of practice.

It's best to start your practice of appreciation with people who naturally elicit a feeling of connection. This might be a dear friend, a mentor, someone who helped you in the past, a family member, or even your pet. Whoever it is, bring them to mind and focus on something positive about them. Let your mind roam. Reflect on their skills and good qualities. Recall warm memories or inspiring moments. Get creative as you clarify all the things you value and respect about this person.

You can also do this as a journaling exercise or a meditative reflection. If you make appreciation journaling or meditation a regular practice, you will find that the skill becomes more automatic. You can even practice this with a partner, taking turns talking about people and sharing what you appreciate about them. It can be especially powerful to do this in your mind when you're going about your day out in the world. As you walk into a room to see someone or pick up your phone to send a quick message, take a moment to notice their positive qualities. It doesn't matter what you notice; it's your perspective that matters. A clear intention to appreciate this person is what matters most.

The skills of kindness and compassion work much the same way. You start where it's easy. Bring to mind someone you care about—whether through journaling, meditation, or conversation—and tap into your desire for this person to be happy, safe, and content. That's kindness. Wish for them to be free from hardship, stress, and suffering. That's compassion.

If you are writing, you can list small acts of kindness that would support this person or things you could do to help them in a difficult time. In meditation, you can repeat caring phrases in your mind, a great way to build awareness and connection at the same time. You can explore kindness and compassion in conversation with a friend or a loved one. The whole point is to immerse yourself in thoughts and feelings that elicit a feeling of connection.

With time and a little practice, feelings of appreciation and warmth will become more and more a part of you. It will also become more natural to express feelings of goodwill when the time is right. That doesn't mean you have to run around telling everyone how much you care about them. Sometimes, it might mean being a good listener or setting your work aside to help someone out. Sometimes, it might mean setting healthy boundaries or giving difficult feedback to someone who needs to hear it. The important thing is that what you do and say will be motivated by care and concern. You will act from a place of connection.

Once you've worked on the skill of connection for a while and have built a strong foundation with people you care about, the next step is to extend these feelings of appreciation outside your circle. This step can be very challenging, but it has the potential to transform our most difficult relationships. This is exactly what happened with John, a friend of ours who was a leader in one of the largest companies in America when we met him.

John was at the top of his game professionally but also struggling to stay on good terms with one of his colleagues. John said their relationship was toxic, and the stress was beginning to spill into his work. His time at the office started to feel miserable. He was not flourishing. When John asked us for advice, we pointed him to the connection practices of appreciation and compassion. We told him about a simple exercise to cultivate appreciation.

"There's only one step, John. It's really simple. All you have to do is notice something positive about your colleague. And do this every day. That's it."

He was incredulous at first. In truth, he didn't want to let go of his harsh judgments. "Why on earth would I want to think warm, fuzzy thoughts about this guy?" he asked. "He's the most annoying person I know!"

"Well, that may be true, but how is your current approach working out for you?" we asked. "Does it feel good to sit around feeling frustrated and resentful? Be honest. How's it going?"

Grudgingly, John decided to give the practice a try.

The following week, John tensed up as soon as he spotted the coworker. But then he remembered the instruction. He noticed his emotional reaction and did his best to find something to appreciate.

He remembered how his colleague spoke lovingly of his two daughters and kept pictures of them on his desk. Not only did this help John appreciate something about his colleague, it also reminded John of his own kids. Immediately, he felt a connection.

This small moment was the beginning of the end of their tense relationship. The fact that John was clearly trying to change the tense dynamic created more space between them. Soon, John's more open stance had a ripple effect, allowing his coworker to make more effort as well. They didn't become best buddies, but the tension and annoyance disappeared. The simple yet difficult step of appreciation erased one of the most stressful elements of John's job.

We all have the capacity to do this at any time. If you are surrounded by family or neighbors with different beliefs or lifestyles or have a coworker who pushes your buttons, notice how it feels to carry resentment and frustration into your interactions. Be honest with yourself and explore what it really feels like. Next, experiment with appreciation. What happens when you focus on their positive qualities instead of all the things you don't like? Maybe they love to garden or have a sweet relationship with their dog. Try it and see if you can soften your judgments. You might not change their political views or the little things that grate on your nerves, but you just might feel a little more connected and a little less judgmental. It's a win-win.

John went straight to one of his more challenging relationships, but generally, it's best to avoid starting with the most difficult person in your life. Begin with someone just outside your circle—a coworker you don't know very well or the person who makes your coffee at your favorite coffee shop. It could be a neighbor you run into on the street or someone you see on your morning commute. You probably won't feel the warm fuzzies when you bring someone like this to mind. That's the whole point. These are people in your "neutral" bucket, people you don't have strong feelings for one way or the other. When you think about them, imagine what it would be like if they really were a close friend or a loved one. They aren't neutral to everyone. They are someone's child. Someone's best friend. Someone out there deeply values and appreciates this person. What might they see when they look at this person?

Keep the exercise light and playful. Reflect on their positive qualities and things you might appreciate about them. If you don't know them very well, use your imagination. Who knows? Maybe they're the funniest person in the world behind closed doors or a world-class banjo player. Wish them well and set an intention to be kind to them when you get the chance or to help them in some small way.

Let's say the person you think about is the guy who picks up the trash in your neighborhood. You might first think about his hard, thankless job and how important it is that someone does this work. Maybe you remember that he always does his job well and doesn't leave a mess behind. He's always on time. He leaves the cans lined up nicely. Even if you don't interact with him directly, you can still do something kind. Maybe you're extra careful to put the trash out in a way that will make his job easier. Perhaps you leave a nice note one day, thanking him for his work so he knows someone appreciates him. If nothing else, simply thinking kind things will prime your mind to do something nice in return should the opportunity arise.

Now, slowly extend your circle further and further. Think about people you don't know: people in other countries, political parties, religions, or groups you disagree with. Eventually, you can experiment with people in your "difficult" bucket. You might not be ready to work with people who have hurt you in the past, but you can experiment with people who rub you the wrong way. Maybe the guy who cuts you off in traffic or the lady who tries to jump ahead in line. This is a lifetime practice.

We often resist the idea of learning to be more kind and caring toward the people and groups we dislike, but most of us would agree that society is in need of a major reset. Our research shows that widening our circles of connection has profound benefits, and not only for ourselves. In our work with teachers, we found that these practices can reduce unconscious bias in the classroom and that the effects don't disappear after training ends. We even found that teachers were more likely to still be teaching three years later, saving school systems the time and money to find and train new teachers. Our world desperately needs more connection, and each of us has a role to play.

When we feel the warm glow of care and compassion, we naturally feel connected to the people in our lives. We also feel uplifted and confident. It's an empowered state of mind. Yet with all the talk of compassion for other people, it can be easy to forget that we need to include ourselves in the circle, too. This might sound a little strange, but the more you feel appreciation and compassion for yourself, the easier it will be to extend it to others.

Right now, in this moment, appreciate yourself for taking the time to learn these skills. It's a wonderful thing! In the same way you notice positive things about others, notice them about yourself. Notice your innate drive to be safe, happy, and content, and nurture it. Recognize the natural movement away from discomfort and hardship. These signals are the innate qualities of kindness and compassion. Practicing self-compassion can be remarkably difficult, but it is a key component of flourishing. We are often our own worst critics, holding ourselves to impossibly high standards. Our minds can be filled with endless running commentary on our flaws and shortcomings. For this very reason, an essential part of practicing this skill is practicing it with yourself. In our often unforgiving world, it is a vital tool to have in your flourishing toolbox.

PRACTICE

Journaling to Nurture Kindness and Compassion

One of the most important parts of cultivating connection is allowing ourselves to truly recognize and experience connection when it happens. Journaling is a great way to take note of the moments of connection in our lives, and by rereading your journal entries you can remind yourself of your connections. Spend a few minutes with the following prompts and try this out for yourself.

Start with kindness. Think back on your life and recall times when someone showed you kindness. It could be something large or small. See what comes to mind, and write a few details down on a pad of paper or in a journal or notebook.

Next, think of times when you were the one being kind. Who was the recipient of your kindness? What did you say, do, or think? Again, write some details down, adding a few sentences about how it made you feel to express kindness.

Now, bring your focus to the present. When have you been on the giving and receiving end of kindness in the past week? It might be something small, like giving someone a tip at a restaurant or taking on an extra task at work. You can keep this light and playful, and see what you come up with.

For the final step, think about the next few days or the upcoming week. You don't have to plan acts of kindness. Instead, plan to notice them when they happen. Think of some specific activities and what kindness might look like in those situations. Jot down some notes that will help you to see kindness more clearly in the coming week.

PRACTICE

The Compassionate Calendar

As time passes, you will begin to see that connection practices enhance your ability to flourish in numerous ways, and you can get more creative with your efforts to cultivate feelings of connection. You can even use connection practices during busy times of stress and feeling overwhelmed to help you slow down and experience moments with others more deeply.

A few years back, Richie's daily schedule had become filled with back-to-back meetings. He was running from one meeting to the next with little time to rest and no space to pause and reflect on how he wanted to interact with the colleagues he was meeting. His interactions felt mechanical, and he started to feel disconnected. At the time, connection practices were a part of his morning meditation routine. He brought different people to mind with kind thoughts and extended compassion to people who got on his nerves. But for whatever reason, his morning practice wasn't linking with his interactions throughout the day.

So Richie decided to try something different. One morning, he looked at his daily calendar to see who he'd be meeting with that day and brought these people into his practice. He thought about each person, one by one. He thought about their work and how he could support them. He took a few moments to appreciate the challenges they were facing and reflected on why they wanted to meet with him. Before he moved on to the next person and the next meeting, he set a clear intention to do his very best to help them in whatever way he could. This short daily exercise made all the difference. No longer going through the motions, Richie was more fully present with each person. Not only did he feel like he was flourishing more at work, but he was also more effective in helping others.

If you'd like to try this practice, here are a few simple steps you can follow:

Each day, pause for a few moments right before you begin your work routine. Take a few calming breaths, center yourself, and form an uplifting motivation to serve the people you work with.

If you use a personal calendar, review each meeting and assignment you have scheduled for the day. If you don't use a calendar, reflect on your day hour by hour and on each activity.

For each meeting, interaction, or activity, think about who you will be seeing and who your work will affect, even if indirectly. Think about the challenges they face and how you might be able to help them.

Form a clear intention to enrich the life and work of each person you think about, using whatever phrases, imagery, or intention-setting works best for you.

Conclude with a moment of appreciation for yourself for taking the time to do this. Then, let go for a few moments. Notice how you feel and take a few more mindful breaths before continuing with your workday.

Your Brain on Connection

Connection is an inner sense of care and kinship with others. This felt sense naturally ripples out and leads to supportive interactions and caring relationships. As we've learned, nurturing qualities like appreciation, kindness, and compassion help us strengthen feelings of connection. Although social emotions are often referred to as "soft skills," hard science shows that these "soft" inner qualities lead to interesting changes in the way our brains function.

The brain networks that underlie our social connections are complex. For instance, take the relationship between empathy and compassion. As we've learned, compassion is critical to our ability to connect. It's also easily confused with its close cousin empathy. Although we often use words like empathy and compassion interchangeably, these are completely different experiences that activate entirely different brain networks. In scientific terms, we think of empathy as the capacity to resonate with another person's emotional state. If a close friend loses their job and shares the bad news, you might feel a little sad and depressed. That's empathy. If that same friend calls you a month later and tells you they got an even better job, you might feel a burst of happiness and joy. That's empathy, too. In both cases, brain networks that mirror what's happening in your friend's brain are activated in your own. If they're in pain, your pain matrix is active. If they're bursting with excitement, it's probably the reward network that's active.

These bursts of empathy can lead in different directions. In the first instance, when your friend lost their job, you might get overwhelmed by sadness. Scientists call this "empathic distress." In some cases, you might have a completely different response. Instead of getting overwhelmed by your feelings, the spark of empathy might transform into warm flames of compassion. Less consumed by your reaction, you are more focused on the motivation to support your friend, express care, and help if you can. This compassionate response activates a completely different network in your brain, what we call the care network. Activity in this network is linked to positive emotions and feelings of connection. Unlike empathic distress, these feelings aren't overwhelming or depleting but uplifting and energizing.

In our research, we've confirmed that compassion works on many levels. It does indeed change how our brains function, but it also impacts how we feel and act in stressful situations. Perhaps even more important, our research shows that our ability to connect is a trainable skill.

In one of our most important studies, we wanted to see if compassion training would get people to act more altruistically, and if it did, whether we would see different patterns of brain activity linked to altruistic behavior. Our colleague Dr. Helen Weng was the lead scientist on this study. She designed an experiment in which 56 research subjects were randomly assigned to receive a 2-week training in either compassion or cognitive reappraisal, a technique from cognitive behavior therapy that teaches people to reframe their interpretations of stressful events to support a healthy emotional response.

Those who received the compassion training were taught to think of specific people and to imagine a time when the person had suffered, to notice their own reactions to the suffering with a nonjudgmental and balanced attitude, and then to repeat caring phrases like "May you be free from suffering. May you have joy and happiness." The subjects trained in cognitive reappraisal were taught 3 strategies for dealing with stressful situations: (1) consider the situation from a new perspective, (2) think about the situation from another person's perspective, such as a friend or a family member, and (3) consider what it would be like a year later if a positive outcome occurred. The cognitive reappraisal group was included as a control treatment. We wanted to have an active comparison treatment that was believable and that required the identical time of engagement.

To see if these two trainings would create unique patterns of brain activity and different social behaviors, Helen used a simple game devised by economists. There were 3 players in the game, one of which was a research subject. The subject would see 1 player, "the dictator," take an unfair amount of money from another player, "the victim." The research subject, who was given $5 at the beginning of the game, was then told they could choose to keep the money or use it to compel the dictator to pay the victim back. The subjects who received compassion training acted more altruistically. They gave nearly 2 times more money than the subjects trained in cognitive reappraisal.

This was not entirely surprising. What was surprising was what happened in their brains. When we put them in the fMRI brain scanner and showed them images of suffering, we saw a diverse set of brain regions activate. We could see that altruistic behavior was linked to what scientists call the mirror neuron system—brain regions linked to empathy, which we mentioned previously. But we also saw a key hub of the brain's executive network come online (the dorsolateral prefrontal cortex, for those of you who might be neuroscience nerds like us). You might remember that this network helps us consciously manage our thoughts, emotions, and impulses. Beyond these two networks, there was also a strong link between the executive network and a region in the care network (and the reward network) that supports positive emotions.

The takeaway message here is that learning to connect will do more than activate your brain's care network. It also seems to strengthen our capacity for self-regulation and increase our tendency to form a healthy response when we encounter suffering, one that helps us stay actively engaged without getting knocked off balance. These findings echo a large and growing body of scientific research that shows how training in appreciation, kindness, and compassion promotes feelings of connection—and this helps us to thrive and flourish.

Limitless Connection

Each of us has limitless, untapped potential for connecting with others. The world's wisdom traditions share a common view that we can extend our circle infinitely, and science is now confirming the value of widening our circle in all directions. As we grow in this way, we will find ourselves in a state of ever more flourishing. Maybe we can't all be the Dalai Lama, but we can establish a steady practice to bring more appreciation, kindness, and compassion into our lives. Imagine what more connection would look like in your life. Imagine letting go of grudges and replacing resentment with compassion and understanding, transforming your apathy into engagement and daily annoyances into opportunities to connect. The inner process of nurturing feelings of connection is one of the most direct and powerful ways to strengthen your ability to flourish.

Connection is available everywhere. The innate capacities we all carry in our hearts, minds, and brains are waiting to be nurtured. This second skill of flourishing doesn't take much, just five minutes a day. Imagine what the world would look like if each of us spent a small portion of each day strengthening our capacity to connect. The world would be a different place, a place we would all want to call home.

Chapter 7

Insight: The Third Skill of Flourishing

The only journey is the one within.

—Rainer Maria Rilke

Laura sat in her car after work, staring at the dashboard in stunned silence. The promotion she had been working toward for the last five years had just been given to someone else. She felt the heat rise in her chest. *How could they overlook me?* she thought. *I've put in the extra hours, delivered results, and stayed committed to the company's vision. Clearly, they don't see my value.*

Over the next few weeks, her mind spiraled into frustration and resentment. She replayed every interaction with her boss, every meeting where she had spoken up—or hadn't. Had she done something wrong? Did they see her as weak? Had they been planning to pass her over all along? The more she ruminated, the more convinced she became that she had failed. Her motivation plummeted, and she began disengaging at work, withdrawing from meetings and avoiding conversations with her colleagues.

Then one afternoon, over coffee with a mentor, she let it all spill out. When she finished, her mentor simply asked, "Have you asked your boss why?"

The question stopped her cold. She had been so consumed by her own assumptions that she hadn't even considered seeking out the truth. That evening, she sat with her thoughts, recognizing how much of her suffering had been shaped by a story she had created in her mind. She made a decision: instead of drowning in speculation, she would get curious.

The next day, Laura walked into her boss's office and asked for a candid conversation. She braced herself for disappointment, but what she heard instead surprised her. Her boss reassured her that she was highly valued—but the role had required international experience, something she didn't yet have. However, there was an opportunity coming up: a six-month global project that could position her for an even bigger leadership role in the future. "If you're open to it," her boss said, "I'd love for you to take it on."

At that moment, the walls of her self-doubt crumbled. The insight was immediate: I spent weeks making up a painful story that had no basis in reality. I assumed rejection when I could have sought understanding. My suffering wasn't caused by the situation itself—it was caused by my interpretation of it.

We've all been there. We jump to conclusions, believing our inner narrative without question. We assume the worst when someone cancels plans. We take a short email as a personal slight. We misinterpret a neutral expression from a friend as judgment. And in doing so, we trap ourselves in unnecessary stress and suffering.

But there's another way. Insight—the ability to see how our thoughts, emotions, and beliefs shape our experience—allows us to break free from these habitual patterns. Laura's moment of insight didn't come from blind luck. It came from a conscious decision to shift from assumption to curiosity, from certainty to open-mindedness.

She saw that her suffering had been fueled not by reality, but by her mind's interpretation of it.

And this is something we can all practice. Instead of being ruled by automatic reactions, we can choose to get curious. We can ask questions instead of assuming answers. We can step back and observe our thoughts before letting them dictate our emotions. And when we do, we give ourselves the space to see more clearly—and to flourish.

The Power of Insight

Insight, the third skill of flourishing, is one of the most powerful skills we can cultivate when it comes to our wandering, ruminating minds. Insight offers us a potent catalyst for personal growth and self-discovery. But what exactly is it? In scientific terms, insight is "the capacity to see how our thoughts, emotions, and beliefs shape the way we see ourselves and the world."

Insight helps us see the whole picture, including how the mind's weather patterns influence perception. When Laura, whose story we shared above, sat in her car after work, she was consumed by thoughts about the promotion she didn't get, and yet she had no idea how much of her suffering came from the story she was telling herself. Her lack of insight in that moment led to weeks of rumination, resentment, and self-doubt. But later, when a mentor's simple question sparked a moment of insight, she saw the situation differently: her assumptions had no solid evidence. This new perspective allowed her to step back and investigate. She could now manage her emotions instead of being ruled by them. Even if her initial fears had been true, insight would have helped her respond wisely rather than spiral into her worst impulses.

Seeing through a faulty interpretation is one form of insight. There are many others. Maybe you're overwhelmed by a difficult problem at work, but when you reflect on the many challenges you've overcome in the past, you can see yourself in a new light. Maybe journaling and reflection help you realize that the sense of identity you've created with your thoughts and memories is an illusion and that there are more subtle dimensions of human consciousness for you to discover. These are just a few of the many variations of insight. All of them are different forms of the experience of seeing something clearly that frees you from an unhealthy or dysfunctional perception.

The ability to see things clearly is profoundly helpful. Insight helps you understand your impulses, reactions, and feelings, which allows you to pause and consider how you want to respond to difficulties at work or with loved ones. With the clear light of insight to guide you, your response will likely be more skillful and wiser, and consequently, your life will improve. Without insight, we're all far more likely to react in ways that perpetuate unhealthy behaviors, thoughts, and emotional patterns.

Insight can help you get to the root of limiting belief systems so you can see how self-defeating thought patterns and emotional habits are getting in the way of reaching your full potential. A flash of insight might help you see that the impulse to lash out when someone cuts you off in traffic won't lead to anything positive or that doomscrolling before bed creates stress when you really want to relax. Insight helps in positive moments, too. When you're in a groove working on an important project, insight can open your mind to new perspectives and ideas. When you're hanging out with friends, insight can help you understand them better and be more empathetic and caring.

Insight is especially helpful and interesting when it comes to how we detect and respond to perceived threats. Humans are terrible at telling the difference between physical and emotional threats or between real threats and the worries that live only in our heads. If you step onto a busy street without realizing a bus is headed your way, your body, brain, and nervous system will immediately react as your fight-or-flight response kicks in and gets you to jump out of harm's way before you even know what happened. Unfortunately, a threat response can also get triggered when a friend or coworker makes an insensitive comment. Your whole nervous system responds as though you're being physically threatened when, in fact, the threat is emotional. Over time, an overactive threat response can turn into a state of chronic stress that exacts a huge toll on your physical and emotional health. In threatening situations, insight can help you see a threat more accurately, allowing you to separate the threat from your interpretations and reactions. This gives you room to respond thoughtfully instead of reacting blindly. When we dig into insight, we can defuse an overactive threat response, even in tricky situations.

Marcus, who used the Healthy Minds Program app, wrote us to share how he used the tools of flourishing, and insight in particular, to improve his marriage. He told us how he was in the kitchen one morning with his wife, and she said something that pushed his buttons hard. "On any other day," he said, "I would have snapped at her, and the whole thing would have spiraled into a pointless argument. But I remembered the idea of getting curious about my habits and reactions, and that took things in a different direction. I noticed that my whole body had tensed up like I was bracing for a physical attack, and my mind was tight, too. It was like my field of vision narrowed. I felt so threatened. But as all this was happening, I knew it was just my biology making an incorrect prediction, so I responded differently. Instead of retaliating, I just let it go. I could see she was tired and irritable, like we both are before our morning coffee. I gave her a hug and told her I loved her before I walked out the door. It was a little thing, but it was so much better than driving to work ruminating about a stupid, pointless argument."

Marcus's experience shows how a moment of insight can change the way a stressful situation plays out. There are many ways we can practice this skill. If you have an anxious temperament, insight can help you notice your fearful thoughts and remind you that they're just mental habits, nothing more than words and images in the mind that aren't necessarily real or true. If you have a short fuse, insight can help you defuse an emotional time bomb before it explodes. Insight can also bring epiphanies. Maybe you realize you are hyperfocused on the negative, which impedes your ability to see anything else. Or maybe, for the very first time, you suddenly see that you've been carrying around an old belief from your childhood that doesn't fit your current reality.

Insight allows you to take a peek at your shadows and inner demons so that they become your greatest teachers. Insight can lead to even more profound changes in the human psyche beyond seeing your mental patterns and emotional habits more clearly and gaining the ability to step back and examine your beliefs and assumptions. When insight is nurtured, it can grow from self-knowledge to self-transcendence. First, you might understand your own mind and how it works. But as you gain more insight, your curiosity will likely grow, and your drive to explore and discover the hidden recesses of your mind may take on a life of its own. As you devote more time and energy to your inner journey, your entire sense of self may begin to change.

Self-transcendence can take many forms. It can manifest as a sense of deep connection with other people, other living creatures, even the entire universe. The boundaries of the self may feel less rigid and defined. The memories and continuous flow of thoughts that usually fill your mind may recede into the background or cease to hold sway altogether. The habitual ways of seeing yourself may ease or disappear and be replaced by an experience of selfhood that is more open, spacious, and less defined by beliefs and concepts. Mystics the world over have tried to capture these experiences in words for centuries. There is broad agreement that transcendent experiences defy description. Simply put, they are ineffable.

In recent years, psychologists and neuroscientists have begun to study insight. One of the pioneers in this area is renowned psychologist Aaron Beck, the founder of cognitive behavior therapy. In a study of people with severe mental illness, he saw that patients who were able to step back and examine their own beliefs and perceptions tended to do better in treatment, while those who were firmly entrenched in their way of seeing did worse. He labeled this capacity "cognitive insight" and developed a scientifically validated questionnaire to measure it. Although Beck's work focuses on helping people with schizophrenia and other psychiatric disorders, we can all benefit from his pioneering research. When we step back to examine our views and question our interpretations, we flourish.

PRACTICE

A Taste of Insight

Moments of insight happen spontaneously all the time, but we can also nurture and strengthen our capacity for self-knowledge and self-discovery through practice. In this practice, you will learn how to use a stressful situation as an opportunity to gain a fresh perspective.

To begin, take a moment to find a comfortable posture and ground yourself with a few slow, calming breaths.

Set an uplifting motivation for your practice by envisioning how this insight meditation might enrich your life and ripple out to benefit others. Imagine that you are bringing more wisdom and insight into the world by taking these few moments to practice.

When you feel ready, bring to mind a stressful situation in your life that could use a fresh perspective. Don't pick the most intense or overwhelming situation. Start with something that feels workable.

As you bring this situation to mind, ask yourself, "What beliefs, assumptions, and expectations do I have about this situation?" Observe what comes to mind without judgment. Bring an attitude of curiosity to your experience as you explore what arises in your mind.

Next, ask yourself, "What would my wisest friend or a mentor say about this situation? What might they see that I am missing?" Again, see what arises in your mind without judgment.

Continue to examine your beliefs and assumptions and see if

> you can look at the situation from a new perspective or uncover reactions that may be distorted or limiting.
> To conclude, note any insights that arose from this reflection. Then, let go and bring awareness into your body as you notice how you feel.
> As you transition into whatever comes next in your day, form a clear intention to explore your expectations and assumptions as you enter each new situation, and apply the skill of self-inquiry in your daily life.

Your Brain on Insight

Insight isn't just getting heavy and deep about all your reactions to what happens in your life. Insight is about seeing things clearly. If you look, you'll notice that you lean on insight all the time. From the moment you wake up in the morning, you are predicting what will happen next. When you roll over to hit snooze on the alarm, you're predicting that it will go off and then come back on a few minutes later. When you turn the bathroom faucet on, you're predicting water will come out. When you have your cup of coffee, you're predicting what it will taste like and how it will make you feel. The number of predictions you make during your morning routine could fill a book.

These small moments of prediction are actually small moments of insight. Your brain is analyzing the data and connecting the dots in experience to prepare you for what might happen next. And usually, you're right. In any given moment, your brain is making countless predictions, and the vast majority are accurate. Our capacity to predict what's coming around the corner is so refined that we don't even notice it. We notice the times when our predictions are wrong precisely because they are comparatively rare. In this way insight is a lot like connection—we tend to notice what's wrong because usually everything is going right. And as with connection, we want to harness and build on the moments of correct insight as a skill.

The bottom line here is that your brain is built for insight. By some estimates, the human brain has roughly 86 billion neurons, and as we discussed in chapter 2, those neurons connect to one another with staggering complexity. There are more than 100 trillion neural connections. That's a whole lot more than the number of stars in the Milky Way. This neural wiring is at your disposal every single moment of your life. It is constantly active, shifting, and changing in a symphony of electrical currents and neurochemical reactions.

The net result is that your brain is continuously learning and growing from experience. It is busy making predictions and adjusting its forecasts. It's a learning machine. In any given moment, your brain is making sense of the world and putting together interpretations. True, some of these interpretations are faulty, but if we learn how to harness this capacity, we can use it to gain insight into ourselves and the world. You could even say that our biological wiring is built for this kind of transformation. We can use all the amazing processing power between our ears to tap our full potential to flourish.

The challenge is that getting it wrong usually feels like failure. We don't recognize and celebrate our insights enough. Instead, we beat ourselves up for falling into bad habits again . . . and again . . . and again. But this dynamic can change if we can recognize our many moments of insight. Making mistakes wakes us up to insight. It's like touching a hot pan. We need the "ouch" to remind us that touching a hot piece of metal is dangerous. Without the pain, we would never change our behavior.

Because of our natural tendency to predict what will happen next, our brains deal with a constant stream of thoughts and images flowing through our minds. This inner monologue is both a blessing and a curse. On the one hand, our ability to weave narratives is a profound gift. It enables us to create meaning, find patterns, and imagine possibilities far beyond our immediate circumstances. This capacity for storytelling has fueled human creativity, innovation, and progress throughout human history. From the earliest cave paintings to the most complex scientific theories, our inner narratives have allowed us to transcend the boundaries of the present and envision what does not yet exist.

Our inner monologue is essential for making sense of our experiences. It helps us integrate new information with the ongoing story of our lives. Through this constant narration, we imbue our lives with purpose, interpret our interactions with others, and (in our better moments) find solace in adversity. Without this ability to weave stories, our existence would be a fragmented series of disconnected moments, devoid of the rich tapestry of meaning that gives depth to the human experience.

Unfortunately, all this creative energy has a dark shadow. The capacity to predict and guess and think and imagine can also be our worst enemy. For example, if you fall behind on an important piece of work, you might get stuck in a loop of toxic rumination, imagining all the bad things that might happen if you can't get it done on time. You might think to yourself: *Oh man! How did I let it get to this point? I'm never going to get this done. Why do I always procrastinate? It's so stupid!* Our inner narratives are often tainted by biases, judgments, and distortions that can sabotage our mental health and well-being. We may find ourselves caught in loops of negative self-talk, ruminating over past failures or catastrophizing about future events. Sometimes, we point the laser beam of negativity at ourselves, and sometimes we focus on others or the whole world. The stories we tell ourselves can become rigid narratives, blinding us to alternative perspectives and keeping us from adapting to changing circumstances.

This persistent inner narration is closely tied to the brain's default-mode network. The default-mode network is that system of interlinked brain regions that becomes active when the mind is not engaged in a specific task. If you stop reading and just sit there for a few moments, this network will become active and trigger the flow of thoughts and inner commentary. This can add to your personal narrative by combining your memories, thoughts, and emotional responses into the subjective storyline of your life, but an overactive default mode can severely disrupt your well-being. If you're caught in a loop of toxic rumination, this network is likely firing on all cylinders. In your best moments, your executive network can help modulate the default-mode network so it doesn't get out of control, but if you struggle to manage your inner narrative, the default-mode network triggers emotional centers of the brain, like the amygdala, creating chronic stress and putting you at risk for a host of mental health issues.

The key to harnessing the power of thoughts and imagination lies in cultivating insight. You don't want to shut off your default-mode network—you want to use it effectively. You want to forge strong connections between the executive network and the default-mode network so that you are in the driver's seat. You can learn to recognize uplifting stories and discard the ones that hold you back by developing the capacity to observe and examine your thoughts without judgment. You can tap into the creative space that gives you fresh perspectives and keep your mind open to new information. With practice, you can create some distance between yourself and the storylines in your mind, which will give you the ability to respond to life's challenges with greater insight and wisdom.

Curiosity and the Practice of Self-Inquiry

The catalyst for cultivating insight is self-inquiry, a very particular form of healthy self-reflection, which is at the opposite end of the spectrum from toxic rumination. Rumination is fueled by negative beliefs, doubts, and judgments, usually about oneself, while self-inquiry invites an open, curious, and nonjudgmental exploration of one's inner experience. Rumination makes judgments; self-inquiry asks questions. Self-inquiry deepens self-knowledge and sparks insights into the many factors that shape our experience of ourselves, our relationships, and the world.

Curiosity is the essential ingredient for transforming our endless stream of mental chatter into transformative self-inquiry. When we're curious, we actively seek new information, even when it challenges our existing views and perceptions. Imagine you've fallen behind on your work, and before you know it, you have more things on your to-do list than you can actually handle. Instead of rolling up your sleeves and getting to work, you get paralyzed and procrastinate or throw yourself into your work like you're doing battle, stressing yourself out in the process.

Ruminating doesn't help in situations like this, though our minds do it anyway. In moments like this, it helps to become curious. Stepping back with some curiosity and open-mindedness will give you a little space from your habitual response. You might ask yourself, *How do I usually respond when I'm overwhelmed with work?* Simply asking this question will likely defuse some of the emotional reactivity surrounding the situation and allow you to examine whether your habitual way of doing things will truly be the best course of action. You might then probe a little deeper:

What automatic thoughts tend to come up when I feel overwhelmed by work?

What feelings and emotions accompany these thoughts?

Do these thoughts and feelings accurately capture the situation? Do they help me see clearly what's happening and how to deal with it?

If not, what am I missing? What might I not be seeing clearly here?

The questions are less important than the willingness to ask. The ability to stay open and curious in stressful moments can short-circuit your habitual patterns and spark moments of insight. It might not change the situation, but it will definitely change the way you handle it, which will allow you to flourish even when a situation is tough.

Pioneering research by our colleague Tania Singer and her team at the Max Planck Institute in Germany showed that self-inquiry does indeed strengthen our ability to regulate our emotional reactions in new and healthy ways. She compared different forms of mental training and found that insight practices lead to different forms of emotion regulation. Self-inquiry was linked specifically to healthy forms of emotion regulation like perspective-taking, planning, and cognitive reappraisal (the process of reinterpreting or reframing a situation to change its emotional impact). In real-world terms, this means that when we learn the skill of self-inquiry, we can examine and better understand our emotional reactions, which leads to more emotional balance and healthier coping strategies.

In one study from our Center, we replicated a growing body of research that shows how cultivating insight and other dimensions of flourishing through meditation training can strengthen connections between the brain's executive network and the default-mode network, the very same set of brain regions that underlies our inner narrative. When we strengthen these connections, we increase our ability to gain insight into unruly thoughts and reduce distracted mind-wandering.

If you tend to replay a painful memory, for instance, a strong connection between your brain's executive and default-mode networks will give you the ability to notice the swirl of thoughts before they hijack your mind and trigger a cascade of emotions. The connection will give you the space to step back and examine your state of mind and see more clearly how your thoughts are shaping your perception. The best news from our research is that we see these benefits in the earliest stages of practice.

It is so easy to be certain. As we age, we become more set in our ways, so the practice of remaining curious takes intention and discipline. There are a number of ways we can remind ourselves to stay curious. One simple way is to link a common experience to an act of curiosity. If you tend to tense your shoulders in moments of stress, bring in a moment of curiosity every time you notice it. Pause for a mindful breath as you relax your shoulders, then ask yourself, *What's going on here? Why am I feeling stressed? How is this showing up in my body, mind, and emotions?* Asking a simple question at the right moment can make a huge difference. Another way to remind yourself to be curious is to place a memorable object or a sticky note where you'll see it.

Holding Beliefs in a Healthy Way

Sometimes, it's not the story we tell ourselves that could use a little insight. Sometimes, it's how we communicate with others. Practicing the skills of flourishing, especially insight, can transform how we express our views and opinions. For example, one area where Cort needed to grow is holding his beliefs in a balanced way. He likes to think of himself as passionately opinionated, but that would be a very generous description. The people who know him best would probably use different adjectives. His parents used to tell him that he would be a lawyer when he grew up, and Cort used to think it was a compliment. Now, with a strong-willed teenage son of his own, he knows exactly what they were talking about.

Cort's "inner lawyer" was on full display in a recent discussion with a good friend over coffee. They started off by catching up on family stuff, but before they knew it, they were in a debate about climate change. Cort held it together for a few minutes as his friend shared his views, but once he started talking about some new legislation that was making its way through Congress, Cort's three decades of meditation practice flew out the window. He lost his patience. "Hold on a minute!" he said indignantly. "You can't possibly believe that! You're an intelligent person. Have you completely lost your mind?"

"I've spent tons of time researching this," his old friend responded sharply. "You're the one who doesn't know what you're talking about."

They went back and forth. Cort's inner lawyer was triggered, and he started citing facts and figures as he built his case. His friend threw conflicting statistics back at him. Each of them tried to sound rational, but to any outside observer, they probably sounded more like bickering fourth-graders. It wasn't long before neither of them was listening to what the other had to say. They were more interested in scoring points than understanding the issue or each other.

This went on and on until something shifted. Cort had a moment of curiosity, which created a little space in his mind. He could see that his mind was caught in an all-too-familiar loop. His body was tense. His mind was churning out thoughts about what he wanted to say next, trying to stay one step ahead in the argument. Along with this heightened awareness came a spark of insight. Cort realized that this loop was keeping him from having a genuine dialogue. He wasn't really listening to what his friend was saying. All his energy was focused on proving him wrong. Cort likes to think of himself as a calm, reasonable, open-minded person, but in this particular moment, he was rigid and dogmatic—things he'd never like to admit about himself.

"Hold on a minute," Cort said, trying to disrupt the blitz. "Let's slow down. I'm sorry for not really listening to you." Hearing these words immediately disarmed his friend. Cort could see the tension in his friend's body release as he dropped his shoulders and took a breath, waiting to hear what Cort would say next.

"I really, really disagree with you. I'm sure you can tell. But I know you have reasons for your views on this. Why don't we start over? I'd like to understand why you see this the way you do."

The conversation did a complete 180. His friend talked. Cort listened. And soon, his friend was asking Cort questions and genuinely listening to what he had to say. The warmth of their connection returned, and with it, mutual respect. Neither of them shifted their views, but they better understood each other's position.

This coffee shop debate was not unique. Our beliefs give our lives meaning, purpose, and direction, but without insight, they can also be a source of alienation and division, in our personal lives and even more so in the fabric of society. This raises the question: How do we get the benefits of a healthy set of beliefs without the nasty hangover of social disharmony? When we find ourselves in a heated debate, how can we stay true to our values without becoming dogmatic and closed-minded? Many things can help, but the ability to stay open and curious is one of the most powerful.

Self-inquiry is the antidote to a closed mind. Instead of walling ourselves off and listening only to our inner monologue, we can practice stepping back to examine our views, beliefs, and the strong emotions that often come with them. We might see that things are more complex than we often believe. There might be more than one side to the argument and more than one valid perspective on a thorny issue. And if we keep our original view, we might do so with more humility and a willingness to listen and learn, however passionately we disagree.

Transform Your Inner Narrative

Awareness practices help us step back and observe our inner narratives without getting swept up in their current. Connection practices like kindness and compassion, especially self-compassion, help us change the content and tone of our inner commentary so the stories we tell ourselves are more caring and supportive and less judgmental. Insight builds on the foundation of awareness and connection by helping us not only observe ourselves and feel connected to others but also deeply explore and understand our inner landscape of memory, emotion, and perception.

In scientific terms, the difference between self-awareness and self-knowledge is captured by the principles of *decentering* and *de-reification*. Decentering, also referred to as defusion, is an important principle in modern psychology, especially in many forms of psychotherapy. It refers to the ability to step back and observe inner experiences like streams of thought and emotional reactions. De-reification involves insight into these same inner experiences but, more specifically, refers to the understanding that our thoughts and emotions are not necessarily true or accurate depictions of reality. Rather, they are mere mental habits.

Take a common experience like getting anxious before giving a presentation or speaking in front of a group. You might find yourself ruminating the moment you wake up in the morning. What if you say the wrong thing or forget your main point? Maybe you'll be incoherent, or the joke you planned will fall flat. A hallmark of the anxious mind is that it narrows our perception so we can only see negative outcomes on the horizon.

If you've been doing your awareness practices, you might suddenly feel like you "wake up" from your thoughts. You spontaneously feel more aligned with the present moment and have a little space to observe the stream of thoughts and images moving through your mind, as if you've found your way to the bank of the river and stepped out of the current onto the shore. This experience of mindful self-awareness is a moment of decentering. You have changed your relationship to your inner narrative. The distance between you and your thoughts will give you more options than when you were caught up in the current. You can be intentional. You might realize that you are being too harsh in your expectations or too unforgiving in your critique of your abilities.

If you've been doing connection practices, you might change your inner narrative's content and tone to one that is more compassionate. *Come on,* you might think, *you'll do great. You've been working on this for weeks. And even if you slip up here and there, who cares? So many people get anxious about public speaking. You're not alone.* In this case, you have brought a kind intention to your inner voice and changed it. You are thinking different thoughts than you were a few moments earlier.

Insight practices will give you a different set of options. Instead of observing all the stories moving through your mind or actively changing them, insight will help you understand them. It might spark the realization that your thoughts are distorting the way you see things. You might see that your line of thinking has you overly focused on the negative. You might even realize where the thoughts are coming from. Maybe you remember a bad experience giving a presentation in school as a child, and that single memory has created a lifelong tendency to assume that any form of public speaking will go poorly. In short, your insight has de-reified the rigidity of your beliefs and expectations.

Pathways to Insight

Insight can be practiced in various ways, each offering unique perspectives and "aha"s that support your flourishing. You don't need to practice all of these methods. Experiment and find the ones that work best for you.

1. Reflective Writing: Writing down your thoughts, feelings, and experiences in a journal can be a very effective way to cultivate insight. The act of writing can help clarify your thoughts and often leads to unexpected insights. Start with a prompt such as "What did I learn about myself today?" or reflect on a specific situation and ask yourself, "Why did I respond the way I did? What can I learn from this experience?" As you write, don't just recount events; delve into the why and how. This practice can uncover patterns in your thoughts and behaviors, leading to valuable insights into your triggers and coping mechanisms.
2. Analytical Meditation: While meditation is often associated with mindfulness and attention, analytical meditation goes a step further by engaging in active inquiry, reflection, and contemplation. Begin by choosing a topic or question you want to explore. Sit in a quiet space, and after calming your mind through a few minutes of breath awareness, direct your attention to the specific situation or topic. Approach it from different angles, asking yourself open-ended questions and observing the responses that arise without judgment. This form of meditation can help break down complex issues into more understandable components, paving the way for insight.
3. Psychotherapy: Psychotherapy provides a structured environment for self-inquiry with the guidance of a trained professional. Therapists can offer different perspectives and ask

probing questions you might not think to ask yourself. This process can lead to significant insights about your thought patterns, emotional responses, and relationship dynamics. Psychotherapy offers a safe space to explore your inner world and uncover insights that can lead to self-discovery and personal transformation.

4. Reflective Dialogue: Conversations with friends, family, or mentors is another avenue for self-inquiry and insight. When you share your thoughts and listen to others, you're exposed to different viewpoints and experiences. Ask open-ended questions and engage in active listening, where you truly hear and consider the perspectives others offer. These dialogues can challenge your preconceptions and prompt reflections that might not occur in solitude.

Each of these practices offers a unique pathway to the cultivation of insight. Whether through the introspective act of journaling, the contemplative space of meditation, the guided exploration of psychotherapy, or the shared understanding of dialogue, each of these methods has the potential to illuminate the depths of your inner world.

PRACTICE

Insight Through Dialogue

Conversation is a wonderful way to learn and practice the skill of self-inquiry. Not only will it deepen your understanding of yourself, but it can also create new bonds and strengthen relationships. You will need a partner for this exercise, with each person taking turns listening and sharing.

To begin, take a moment to decide who will share first, then set a clear intention to stay open, curious, and supportive throughout the entire exercise.

The person sharing starts the dialogue by describing a meaningful or transformative experience. Try to provide as much detail as possible. What happened? Who was involved? What do you remember most vividly?

Next, the listener can ask questions to spur further investigation: Why was this experience so transformative? What did you learn about yourself? What new insights and self-knowledge did it lead to?

Continue to examine and reflect on the situation together. The listener should mainly hold space and occasionally ask a supportive question. There is no need to comment on or judge what the sharer offers. You can take as long as you like through further rounds of sharing and questioning.

For the second step, the listener prompts the sharer to apply the shared insights to a new situation: What's going on in your life these days? Are there any situations where you could apply these

> insights? How might this transformative experience shed some new light on your current life and experience?
>
> Again, take turns listening, asking, and reflecting.
>
> Once the sharer is done, switch roles and repeat the process.
>
> At the end of the practice, share any final thoughts and thank each other for sharing insights and supportive listening.

Masters of Insight

As we've explored, insight can happen through journaling, simple reflection, or conversation, but with practice, it can become natural and spontaneous. Think of a time when you had a sudden epiphany about your life, a breakthrough, or a super-creative insight. Practicing insight sets the stage for this to happen far more often. And practice helps you sustain and savor those breakthrough moments. Becoming more proficient in the skill of insight will not only enhance flourishing but also change the way your brain functions.

We've been privileged to study the brains of "masters of insight," advanced practitioners who devote their lives to exploring subtle states of consciousness and the complex inner world of thought, emotion, and perception. In the early 2000s, we worked with a small group of such "Olympian" meditators at our brain imaging facilities at the University of Wisconsin–Madison. We wanted to see how insight, in particular, showed up in their brains, so we examined them during different styles of practice, measuring the electrical activity in their brains with an EEG.

We discovered a unique pattern of brain activity during periods of deep insight, especially when insight was linked with compassion. Normally, we don't see a signal with the naked eye. It takes months of complex data processing and statistical analysis to get the final results. But on this particular day, the data were so pronounced we could see the signal in real time. We were shocked. We were so surprised that we literally spent the next year investigating and ruling out the many less-interesting alternative explanations for this finding, such as it being caused by various types of artifact that can easily intrude in measurements of brain electrical activity. For example, we know that activity from facial muscles can masquerade as brain activity as it overlaps in the frequency of oscillations. There are specific tests we conducted to differentiate between muscle activity and brain activity, and we were able to confirm that our finding was produced by the brain and not by facial muscles. After we were able to eliminate all the alternative explanations, we concluded that we were witnessing a new scientific discovery: the first scientifically documented occurrence of individuals who could induce and sustain states of gamma activity by generating inner states of insight and understanding.

The brain exhibits what are commonly known as brain waves, rhythmic patterns of neural activity that fluctuate depending on our inner mental states. Delta oscillations are slow wave patterns that occur during deep, dreamless sleep, while alpha waves are more rapid and occur when we are resting and relaxed. On the other end of the spectrum are gamma oscillations. Gamma waves are extremely rapid, operating at a frequency between 30 and 100 Hz, and are linked to "aha" moments and experiences of insight. If you are puzzling over a difficult problem and suddenly come up with the answer, you are likely producing a burst of gamma oscillations. These are moments when previously unconnected concepts or data points suddenly click into a unified new understanding. Occurrences of gamma activity are typically extremely brief. When they happen, there is a sharp spike of gamma activity followed by a rapid return to baseline.

The masters of insight we were studying showed periods of sustained gamma activity that had never been seen. Things got even more interesting when we talked to them. Keep in mind that these were very advanced practitioners. Each of them had meditated more than 30,000 hours over the course of their lives. When we asked them what they were experiencing during these periods of sustained gamma activity, at first they didn't say much, but eventually they opened up and told us about the practice they were doing—a very advanced practice that combines compassion with deep insight and self-knowledge. They described an experience of looking into the very nature of consciousness, one that produced a state of effortless yet total presence infused with boundless warmth and compassion radiating out like the rays of the sun.

Our subjects were all practitioners of a specific Tibetan Buddhism lineage famous for its teachings on "pure awareness." This tradition, known in Tibet as Dzogchen, or the "Great Perfection," contains step-by-step instructions for generating insight. Practices often focus on a direct, experiential examination of conscious awareness, particularly on the question of whether the objects of awareness are truly separate from the awareness experiencing them. This might sound like a strange topic to explore, but those who do these practices hold that the unconscious belief in a self that is completely independent of everything it experiences is the most basic form of ignorance, and one that is the very root of the chronic stress and suffering that permeate our lives.

However esoteric, the point here is that these advanced practitioners had mastered the cultivation of insight. Observing these virtuosos of flourishing in action was itself a transformative experience. They were radiant despite the stress of endless cognitive tasks and the cold, sterile environment of the brain imaging laboratory. Although few of us will ever reach the levels of inner mastery these masters exhibited in our research, they showed us just how much untapped potential exists within each one of us.

Insight for the Rest of Us

The gamma activity findings were inspiring and left us with an important question: What about the rest of us? Do we have to spend thousands of hours cultivating insight to flourish, or will a few minutes a day do?

Fast-forward to 2016, when we received a piece of advice from the Dalai Lama that changed the course of our research. We had recently identified the key skills of flourishing that comprise the Healthy Minds Framework. We were especially intrigued by the data that showed how central insight is to well-being and flourishing. At the same time, we needed to figure out how to translate the research into a practical skill and include it in our Healthy Minds Program.

As luck would have it, the Dalai Lama was visiting Madison that year for a special event at the Center for Healthy Minds. The timing was perfect. We had several questions we wanted to ask him about insight.

At our meeting, Richie began, "Your Holiness, we've developed a new scientific framework that highlights four key skills of flourishing, but we want to do more than publish data. The world is experiencing a mental health crisis that is getting worse by the year. It's not enough to do research anymore. We need to do something. Our plan is to translate our research into a tool that anyone can use to strengthen the four skills of flourishing and that scientists can use to better understand how flourishing can be cultivated."

As Richie went on to explain that mindfulness was quickly becoming a mainstream topic and that interest in meditation and other forms of practice was exploding, the Dalai Lama suddenly leaned forward in his seat. "Mindfulness is not enough," he said firmly. "We need compassion. We need wisdom. We need to understand the nature of reality."

This is exactly what we were hoping to hear. It supported our new framework and the idea that flourishing has different dimensions, all of which play a unique role in our mental health and emotional well-being. But we were also surprised to hear him talk about understanding the nature of reality. Buddhist practices focus on exploring the deeper reality underlying our beliefs and perceptions, but we didn't want our new framework to be focused on a religious belief system. We couldn't see a clear path forward.

"How can people learn to have more insight?" Cort asked. "Should we include Buddhist principles like impermanence and interdependence in our new training program?"

"No, no . . . don't do that," the Dalai Lama said, shaking his head. "That's Buddhist business! You should take the insights from modern science and teach people how to use analytical meditation to experience the insights directly, not just as intellectual theories and information, but as ideas they can use to train their minds."

The Dalai Lama had just given us the blueprint for building the insight module of the Healthy Minds Program.

"So we take the insights from scientific research and then use insight-based practices like analytical meditation to examine our experience, using these insights as a basis for our exploration. Is that it?"

"Yes, exactly. But you have to use the right kind of practice. Shamatha meditation," he said, referring to the awareness practices that form one of the two main categories of Buddhist meditation, "is great for training attention and becoming more mindful, but it's not enough on its own. You also need insight, and for insight, you need analytical meditation."

This was a bold new idea: combine the insights of modern science with the ancient technology of self-inquiry and inner exploration. This was different from simply doing research on mindfulness meditation.

Building on this advice from one of the great living embodiments of wisdom, we did eventually combine science and contemplative practices in the Healthy Minds Program, including a whole course of step-by-step training in insight. Hundreds of thousands of people have learned the skill of self-inquiry through the program. Many have reached out to us and shared stories from their personal journeys. We are only beginning to understand what happens in the minds and brains of people who practice this skill, but it's clear that even a few minutes a day can help us cultivate more wisdom.

Together, awareness, connection, and insight are a potent combination for transforming the inner experiences that shape our sense of self. Instead of triggering loops of automatic thoughts and emotional reactions, old habits and outdated beliefs slowly spark empathy and self-knowledge as they lose their power over us. You will not only understand yourself better but also other people. With the skill of insight, you are more likely to find yourself flourishing.

Chapter 8

Purpose: The Fourth Skill of Flourishing

When you do things from your soul, you feel a river moving in you, a joy.

—Rumi

In 2001, Cort began his first year living in Tibetan refugee settlements in Kathmandu, Nepal. Kathmandu is nestled in the rolling foothills of the Himalayas. On a clear day, you can see the peak of Everest off in the distance from the valley rim. The city sprawls across the valley floor, with nearly 1.5 million people crowded together in a patchwork of concrete buildings and homes with earthen walls and thatched roofs. Kathmandu boasts some of the most distinctive architecture in Asia, including the towering Buddhist monuments of Boudhanath and Swayambhu and the classic architecture in Patan, where the most famous craftspeople of the Buddhist world have lived and worked for centuries.

When the Tibetans fled their homeland during the Communist invasion in 1959, many, including the Dalai Lama, settled in northern India, but many more landed in Kathmandu. Boudhanath was and is home to one of the largest communities of Tibetans outside Tibet.

Centered on the famed Boudhanath stupa—that massive reliquary with legendary eyes gazing off in all four directions—the Tibetans and local Nepalis have created a maze of tiny shops, teahouses, and hole-in-the-wall restaurants, catering to the endless flow of tourists and the throngs of pilgrims who travel from across the world to pay homage to the ancient Buddhist monument. The smell of incense is inescapable, and everywhere you look are maroon-clad monks and nuns and ordinary Tibetans of all ages, thumbing their bodhi-seed malas as they mutter mantras and prayers.

When Cort arrived at Boudhanath, he couldn't help but notice how joyful everyone seemed to be. There was a sense of ease in the people he met, and the pace of life seemed much more relaxed than in the West. This was not at all what he expected. He had imagined poverty and misery, with refugees deprived of so many of the things most of us take for granted and struggling to survive. But the reality was entirely different. The people he met were indeed very poor by any objective standard. Huge extended families lived together in tiny dwellings. Mothers hawked trinkets on the streets, eking out a meager income, with their small children playing nearby. Newly arrived refugees in tattered clothes filled the streets, having just made the arduous trip over 18,000-foot Himalayan passes. Yet the air was filled with laughter. Many people had a sparkle in their eyes, as if they had figured out some life secret most of us have never learned.

The Tibetans' relaxed lifestyle and joyful ease were a sharp contrast to the life Cort had grown up with. He was used to rushing from one activity to the next and a to-do list that never ends. He even viewed his meditation practice as yet another activity to accomplish each day. The contrast helped him see that the modern world's endless rush comes at a cost. From the time we are small children, we are taught to perform, set goals, and measure our self-worth by what we achieve and possess. Even if we don't buy into the capitalistic ethos of the modern world, it's impossible to escape the twenty-first century's obsessive energy. We may not always know what we're rushing toward or why, but we keep pushing through, harder and harder, without any true connection to what we're working for. For many of us, the frenetic energy is so pervasive we don't realize there's another way to live.

Without the space to step back from the rat race of modern life, we have precious little time or energy to reflect on what truly matters to us. We deprive ourselves of the opportunity to clarify a sense of purpose that brings meaning to our lives and to reflect on what we do each day to ensure we are spending our time wisely. The Tibetans have created that space to connect to purpose each day, and it showed.

Seeing them re-create their lives in exile shifted Cort's perspective on the important role purpose plays in our ability to flourish. Despite the objectively desperate circumstances of living as refugees, the strength of spirit and joyful presence of the Tibetans Cort met was palpable. As he immersed himself in his new surroundings and learned the Tibetan language, Cort began to understand why. Their strong sense of community was certainly part of what allowed them to flourish, but more than anything else, it was the fact that they lived with a sense of purpose.

As a community and culture, Tibetans are led by a deep and abiding commitment to "benefiting all beings." They carry this sense of purpose into everything they do. Cort observed this many times over during his first few months in Nepal. Tenzin, a young man who taught Cort conversational Tibetan, explained: "We Tibetans believe that our own happiness is linked to the happiness of all living beings, so we always do our best to help others. We try to ease their suffering if we can or, at the very least, not do anything harmful. Trying to help all beings is part of our culture."

The phrase "for the benefit of all beings" was a constant refrain, and small acts of kindness and generosity were everywhere. Cort could see it in the way the Tibetans respected and cared for the elderly, dropped what they were doing to help someone, and shared money and belongings with those in need, although many had precious little to share. In simply observing how they lived, Cort could see that this pervasive sense of purpose was almost like a superpower. They didn't need to think or talk about their purpose. They lived it. Their spontaneous care for the world even extended to living creatures to whom most of us wouldn't give a second thought. Countless times, Cort witnessed someone stop on a busy street to move a bug so it wouldn't get stepped on or to pick up a worm after a monsoon rain and put it on some dirt so it wouldn't die. It was completely natural and spontaneous. People, even little kids, took time to care for the world and everything in it. This core purpose seemed to be hardwired into their cultural DNA.

This isn't meant to say that Tibetan culture is some utopia where everyone is perfectly selfless and working for the greater good. Like all societies, they have their fair share of problems, and not everyone fully embodies this cultural sense of purpose. Nevertheless, their shared sense of purpose is a central force in Tibetan culture that shows up in many areas of life.

The more time Cort spent in Nepal, the more he started to wonder about his purpose and whether he embodied it. He was living a spartan life at the time, renting a single room on a dusty dirt road for $30 a month. The building had no hot water, so a hot shower was not an option. The room was tiny, with no furniture save for a rickety old desk and chair he bought for $10 and the blue foam mat he slept on, the only thing between his worn sleeping bag and the cold cement floor. Despite his modest dwelling without the creature comforts he was used to, Cort was flourishing. It slowly dawned on him that what made it possible for him to flourish was that he was indeed living with a strong sense of purpose. It wasn't that he was doing something profound to solve world hunger or end the climate crisis. It was more a feeling that he was genuinely doing his part. He was contributing to the world in a way that felt beneficial. At the end of a long day, he often thought, *That was a day well spent!* In his interactions with others, his work translating ancient meditation manuals, and even how he spent his free time, his aim, his purpose, was clear.

The Power of Purpose

Why is life sometimes filled with meaning yet dull and mundane at other times? At first glance, it might seem that it all comes down to what you're doing. If you're doing interesting or fun things, life is great—but if you're not, well, you're out of luck. If you look a little closer, though, you will see that things are more complex. While it's certainly true that we flourish when we are with people we love and doing things we love, there are also times when that is not the case. Sometimes we flourish in the most challenging situations.

Consider the life of Nelson Mandela. Most of us remember him as the inspiring world leader who ended apartheid in South Africa, but during his life he endured tremendous hardship on his journey to becoming a transformative world leader. He was unjustly imprisoned for decades and lived in the most abject conditions, with little food and clothing and often sleeping on a cement floor. Yet despite the overwhelming adversity he experienced, he flourished and emerged from prison a transformed man.

Mandela was certainly not with the people he loved doing the things he cared about while imprisoned. So what made it possible for him to flourish during those challenging years? His writings make clear that he was driven by a deep sense of purpose, one that gave him the inner strength to deal with challenges most of us could not imagine. He wrote about his prison cell as a place of growth and self-transformation and his confinement there as an opportunity to cultivate the very best in himself so he would be ready to serve others when the time was right. His values and principles coupled with his motivation to leave the world a better place than he found it gave him the inner resources to deal with unimaginable hardship.

Mandela's story illustrates how a sense of purpose is key to the art of flourishing. A clear and meaningful sense of purpose energizes and inspires us, even when life is difficult. It lights the way and helps us be the best version of ourselves. It gives us perspective and helps us develop our full potential. A sense of purpose can lead us toward the light at the end of the tunnel when we're on the verge of giving up, and it can spur us to learn and grow from the challenges we face.

What Is Purpose?

So what exactly is purpose? In scientific terms, we think of purpose as "a clarity about our deeper aspirations and guiding principles and the ability to apply them in daily life." For example, if you are a teacher, your deepest aspiration might be for every student to learn and grow. That guiding principle could be your North Star, the motivation that inspires you in your work and helps you deal with all the stress and hardship of your profession. Along with your professional purpose, you might have different motivations in your personal life. Maybe you're passionate about reducing the impact of climate change or supporting the arts in your community. Maybe you simply want all the people in your life to feel cared for. You don't need one single, life-defining purpose. You can have many.

Having a sense of purpose starts with getting clear about what really matters in life. When you're teaching your fifth class of the day and none of the kids are listening to you, not knowing why you are there or chose this profession won't support the kids or you in making the day feel meaningful. If you can remind yourself why you are doing your job, it will direct you and give you the energy to keep going. Knowing your purpose will put your problems and setbacks into perspective.

But knowing your purpose isn't enough. You also need to embody your purpose. It needs to manifest in what you say, do, and think. For instance, you're in the classroom and crystal clear about your deeper motivation. You remind yourself why you're there in the first place and remember that you want to be kind and caring to all your students. This inner clarity will help, but if your actions don't line up with your guiding sense of purpose, you might feel stressed out—at the very least, you'll feel some inner tension from the disconnect between your beliefs and your actions.

At first glance, clarifying your purpose in life might sound like a heavy, soul-searching exercise, but a purpose can come in many shapes and sizes. Your morning routine might be informed by a deep-rooted belief in the importance of physical health and hygiene, and that might be linked to your aspiration to live a long, healthy life so you can be here to serve your community and care for your loved ones. At work, you might be driven by an entirely different purpose. Maybe you're guided by the wish that the communities your company serves are enriched by the work you do, or maybe you simply want your coworkers to have a harmonious, supportive work environment. When you're with family and friends, your purpose might be that they feel loved and cared for. The point is not to find a single purpose that defines your entire life but rather to shift your perspective on the things you do to see the deeper purpose that is already there, buried beneath the surface.

Finding a sense of purpose can be a light, playful exercise. You can experiment with different perspectives and see what feels right. Let's say you struggle to feel a sense of purpose at work. You may view your job as a paycheck and nothing more. The idea that there is some profound purpose underneath it all may feel foreign or flat-out wrong. But dig a little deeper. Why do you want the paycheck in the first place? Maybe you want to get your finances in order to pay down your debt. And why would you want that? The debt may feel like a burden, and you want to remove the stress. You want to be debt-free because you'll feel more content. So all your hard work for that paycheck is part of a larger vision: you want to be in control of your destiny. Every moment of work is part of that vision, leading you closer to that goal, no matter how distant it may feel at times. The key here is to explore your perspective until you find something that feels meaningful and motivating. With time and a little patience, you will see that there are many layers of purpose in every situation and activity.

PRACTICE

A Taste of Purpose

Purpose is a skill you can cultivate, like awareness, connection, and insight. You can clarify what matters most in your life and experiment with new ways to stay connected to your guiding sense of purpose from moment to moment. Try this short practice to get a feel for it:

To begin, take a moment to sit in a comfortable posture and ground yourself with a few slow, calming breaths.

When you feel ready, bring to mind someone who inspires you, someone who in some way represents the best of humanity. It doesn't have to be someone you know personally. It can even be someone from the past.

Purpose: The Fourth Skill of Flourishing

Reflect on why this person inspires you. What is it about them? Is it a quality they have? Is it how they live their lives or something they do for others? See if you can pinpoint what resonates with you about this person.

Now, see if you can distill this into one guiding purpose. Maybe they selflessly help everyone in their community gain access to a quality education, or they brighten the world with their commitment to the arts. See if you can capture the guiding sense of purpose behind their actions.

Once you've clarified this purpose, step back and look at your own life. How do you embody this purpose? Find specific examples and situations in which you embody this same sense of purpose.

Now, think about the next few days. How might you embody this purpose in your life? Again, think of specific people and situations and set a clear intention to bring this purpose to life in these situations.

To conclude, bring your awareness back to this moment. Notice any feelings or sensations in your body, without any judgment. Take a few slow, calming breaths and transition into whatever you are doing next as you explore new ways to bring this sense of purpose into your daily routine.

You can do this practice in any situation. Experiment with different ways of viewing the activities in your daily routine. What would it look like to view a trip to the grocery store as an opportunity to enrich the lives of the people you see and interact with? What would it look like to see stressful situations as opportunities to model your belief in the power of continuous learning and growth? The skill of purpose is best applied in the small moments of everyday life. With time, even the most mundane situations can be transformed into meaningful moments.

The Science of Purpose

The topic of purpose looms large in the scientific literature about what allows us to feel a sense of well-being. In an influential framework created by our colleague Carol Ryff, purpose is identified as one of six dimensions of well-being, alongside self-acceptance, positive relationships, personal growth, personal autonomy, and environmental mastery (referring to the ability to manage one's life and circumstances effectively). Someone who scores high on purpose in this framework has meaningful goals and a sense of direction. They hold beliefs that imbue their life with a sense of purpose and meaning. Someone who scores low in this area does not see their past or current life as meaningful. They likely lack meaningful aspirations and goals or a direction that lends meaning to their personal journey.

A wealth of research spanning five decades reveals that a strong sense of purpose acts as a superpower, enhancing both mental health and physical well-being. When life feels meaningful and goal-directed, we thrive—experiencing greater cognitive function, emotional resilience, and even better financial health. Conversely, lacking purpose leaves us vulnerable to psychological distress and a range of mental health challenges.

Purpose also plays a crucial role in physical health and longevity. Higher levels of purpose are linked to fewer heart-related issues and a lower risk of stroke. The benefits extend to brain health as well. Recent findings from our Center show that a strong sense of purpose supports healthy aging, particularly in brain regions tied to learning and memory that are susceptible to stress. These insights highlight the potential for purpose-driven interventions to enhance both individual well-being and public health.

Finding Purpose in Adversity

Consider how purpose might show up in your life. Say you just experienced the end of a long-term relationship you thought would last a lifetime. The breakup wasn't just emotionally devastating—it disrupted your sense of the future, your social circle, and even your living situation. If you frame this solely as a personal failure or rejection, you might find yourself replaying conversations looking for where things went wrong, avoiding mutual friends to escape reminders of your ex-partner, and creating narratives that minimize the relationship's value to protect yourself from pain. Your trust in others—and yourself—might erode, making new connections seem risky and undesirable.

Now, imagine a different scenario. What if this heartbreak becomes a catalyst for deeper self-understanding? You begin to reflect: This isn't the outcome I wanted, but what might this experience be teaching me about relationships and myself? You start to recognize patterns in how you connect with others—perhaps you've prioritized taking care of others' needs while neglecting your own, or maybe you've struggled to communicate your deepest values. You might discover that the relationship's end creates space for friendships that had been neglected, or for family bonds that need renewal. Perhaps you even find yourself able to offer wisdom and comfort to others navigating similar losses. With this perspective, you've connected your personal pain to a broader purpose of authentic connection. The grief remains real, and there will still be moments of profound sadness, but you're no longer defined solely by the loss. Instead, you're engaged in the meaningful work of exploring the things that give life meaning.

Purpose helps us cope with adversity. Adversity can leave us with emotional scars that linger for years, even decades. We might end up with post-traumatic stress disorder, a condition that locks us into a feeling of being on guard and seeing danger around every corner. But we can learn and grow from adversity instead, and purpose is a key ingredient in helping us recover with more ease.

Richie's experience of shepherding his son through a difficult adolescence taught him powerful lessons about his commitment to family and how a shared sense of purpose holds families together in tough times. He had no choice but to take stock of his life and decide what was most important. Richie's passion for research and his dedication to his career had always been central in his life, but during this period, it wasn't the most important thing. Caring for his family was his North Star, which meant other priorities in his life, even science, needed to take a back seat.

A clear sense of purpose gives us a broader perspective on the struggles we face in life. Take the experience of Maria, a nurse we met through one of our research studies in a local hospital. From a young age, Maria felt called to care for others and eventually became a nurse. Over her twenty-year career, she developed strong bonds with her patients and their families as she guided them through illnesses, injuries, and the highs and lows of the human experience. But her world was upended when she was forty-two and diagnosed with an aggressive form of cancer. The grueling treatments left her physically and emotionally drained. There were days when she could barely summon the energy to get out of bed, let alone carry on with her work as a nurse. Maria felt her sense of purpose slipping away and, with it, her identity.

During one hospital stay, a young patient named Emma noticed Maria's hairless head and asked if she was also battling cancer. The two formed an immediate connection. Maria told us how she could see the fear, resilience, and hopefulness in Emma's eyes—the same emotions Maria had witnessed countless times in her patients throughout her career as a nurse—and how her purpose became clear again in that moment. She was put on this earth to help people through unimaginable difficulties with her empathy, strength, and compassion. Her own health struggle allowed her to relate to patients on an even deeper level. She had a unique perspective that could provide tremendous hope and reassurance. Even though she was now a patient, Maria discovered she could help other patients in new ways. She struck up friendships with others who were struggling with cancer and did her best to support them.

Maria's life purpose wasn't just about being a nurse but someone who eases suffering in whatever way they can. This driving sense of purpose gave her the courage and resilience to continue fighting her battle with cancer. She was needed and had too much important work left to do. Eventually, Maria recovered and returned to her work with renewed passion and a wider perspective.

Having a sense of purpose can transform major life challenges into opportunities for growth and self-discovery. Adversity can serve as a catalyst that prompts us to reevaluate our life priorities and values. A serious illness, an unexpected breakup, a lost job, a serious accident, all of these circumstances can spur self-reflection that strengthens our sense of purpose, prompting us to deepen our relationships and reconnect with what truly matters in life with a renewed sense of direction and fulfillment.

Meaning in the Mundane

Do you remember sitting in school as a kid and watching the clock as the seconds ticked by in slow motion? All you wanted was for class to end. Your teacher droned on about tests and homework. You exchanged bored glances with your friends. Every minute seemed like an eternity. For many of us, school was a meaningless exercise created by well-intentioned but clueless adults. Does getting an education need to be this way? Research suggests that it doesn't.

A series of studies from a team of Stanford University scientists shows that brief reflections can reframe mundane situations—in this case, the situation of an educational setting. Their hypothesis was simple: if kids see their educational journey in light of their most important values and guiding principles (the foundation of purpose), they'll do better in school.

To put their idea to the test, the researchers randomly divided more than 500 middle schoolers into two groups. Most of the students were from low-income families and backgrounds that put them at risk for poor educational outcomes. Many were from immigrant families where no one had gone to college.

Once the students were divided into two groups, all the students did a series of brief exercises, roughly fifteen minutes each, spread out over a few years. The students in one group wrote about their most cherished personal values and principles, while the second group wrote about neutral topics, like their afternoon routine or values they considered unimportant. Some students did only a single reflection while others did as many as eight, but most did five or six. The scientists wanted to see if a few short reflections could make a real difference in these kids' lives. It was a tall order. The deck was already stacked against these at-risk kids. The interventions were brief and spread out over the students' middle school years.

When the data came back, the results were astounding. Students in the control group, who were asked to reflect on meaningless topics, felt less belonging in school. But the students who reflected on their core values had a different experience. In the first part of the study, which tracked immigrant and low-income Hispanic students, these students were more likely to engage in a college-readiness track than a remedial-learning track. In the second part of the study, which focused on middle- and low-income Black students, students who received the purpose intervention were more likely to enroll in college and attend more selective colleges.

The most surprising thing about the results was that these positive outcomes happened *years later*. In the first part of the study, students could take a college-readiness track two years later. The second part of the study showed an even bigger gap. The students who went to college did so seven to nine years after the intervention. The scientists had discovered something quite amazing: an hour or two of self-reflection can instill a sense of purpose that stays with kids for years, transforming how they see themselves and improving real-world educational outcomes.

This pioneering research tells us a few important things about purpose and our ability to flourish. First, it clearly shows that purpose can be learned and practiced with a relatively small investment of time. Second, it demonstrates that bolstering a sense of purpose does more than make life feel meaningful and rewarding; it also improves hard-nosed objective metrics like college enrollment rates. This series of studies elegantly shows that how we feel affects the decisions we make and the way we behave—and in turn, the decisions we make further shape the way we see ourselves. In other words, flourishing is more than a state of mind. It affects everything in our lives, from our mental health to our immune system's functioning and even our decisions during major life transitions.

If reflecting on what truly matters in life can affect huge decisions like choosing to go to college, imagine how it might affect us as a daily ritual. What would this look like in your life? How would it feel to reflect on one of your deepest aspirations when you wake up each morning or look back at the end of each day to find moments that reflect an important purpose? What if you view stressful situations as opportunities to embody the principles that inspire you and mundane daily routines as periods for self-reflection? We can connect to purpose anytime and anywhere. When we do, it has the potential to transform our perspective and imbue our lives with a profound sense of meaning.

Nourish Your Mind

Unfortunately, the world is not doing us any favors these days when it comes to connecting with a sense of purpose. We are bombarded with news and information, knocking us off the course of what matters to us. It's like we're feeding our minds a steady diet of choices and junk food. Imagine spending a few days eating nothing but potato chips and soda. How would you feel? Now imagine you ate only junk food for a whole year or an entire decade. Every aspect of your life would be affected. You'd have less energy to get through the day, your body would lack the nutrients it needs to fight off illness, and your mood and mental health would take a hit as well.

Your mind works the same way. Information is like food, and the information you're feeding your mind can have real impacts on your daily life. The podcasts you listen to, the books and articles you read, the topics you discuss with your friends, the apps you use—it's all information. You are feeding your mind constantly, and what you choose to feed your mind can help you stay connected to your purpose or make it harder. In other words, staying connected to purpose does take some grit.

Unfortunately, we can't always control the mental food that shows up on our collective dinner table. Cultural forces can limit those choices, and our information diet has steadily become more toxic over the past century.

One way to understand a culture is to analyze the things it produces, such as its stories, songs, and commercials. These things hold important clues about the dominant messages that are influencing our lives at a societal level. Dr. Pelin Kesebir, one of our brilliant colleagues at the Center for Healthy Minds, and her twin sister, Dr. Selin Kesebir, who is also a social psychologist, set out to examine cultural trends in the United States. They came up with the idea of looking at books, thinking that influential trends in society would show up in what people write. They were specifically interested in ideas related to moral excellence and good character, things like cultural values and ideas people find meaningful.

Pelin and her sister analyzed millions of digitized American books from the twentieth century to see how frequently people used terms like *virtue, honesty, compassion, wisdom*, or *tolerance*—words linked to values, purpose, and meaning. Their analysis revealed that from 1900 through 2000, people used these words less and less. For example, the use of the word *virtue* steadily declined over the course of the century. It had a brief resurgence in 1945, right around the end of World War II, but other than that, it's pretty much been downhill, with a low point in the mid-1980s. They also saw that words indicating care and concern for others, such as *thoughtfulness, helpfulness,* or *politeness*, dropped more than 50 percent over the century. The same was true of virtues related to humility, modesty, and gratitude. And then, some specific virtues like kindness dropped almost 70 percent. Overall, there was a decline in how frequently people wrote about words like these in the twentieth century.

There is obviously more to culture than what we write in books, but if we assume that millions of books reflect a trend, then it's safe to assume the quality of our information diet has been in steady decline, at least as far as values and purpose are concerned. The brain food we have access to has been getting increasingly unhealthy. And that's just based on literature. We haven't even factored in the impact of the internet, the twenty-four-hour news cycle, or social media.

In the face of this onslaught, cultivating a resilient, healthy mind is more challenging than ever but far from impossible. We need to feed our minds a healthy diet that supports a sense of purpose, and we need to nurture the best in ourselves by creating daily rituals, moments in our day when we pause to reflect on what inspires and motivates us to reconnect with the aspirations that give our lives meaning. Purpose is not something we lack. It is lying just below the surface in almost any situation. We just need to practice the skill.

Purpose Is a Skill

Feeling a sense of purpose in life is an innate capacity. Whether we recognize it or not, we all have core values that can shape our deeper aspirations into a sense of purpose. The skill is to bring our deepest values and aspirations to the surface of our conscious awareness so we can see them clearly and keep them in mind as we navigate the peaks and valleys of life.

Practicing this skill involves three steps. They can be done anytime that your life or whatever you are doing feels meaningless or disconnected from a sense of purpose that feels inspiring or nourishing. Reflecting on the following points as you transition between activities can be especially helpful since these are the natural "gaps" in our day when we may have a few moments to step back and consider our perspective. If you have time, you can pause and practice more formally, but since this isn't always realistic, it can be especially helpful to create a simple ritual of bringing the following three steps to mind for just a few moments as you start something new. The key is to experiment and see what works best for you. The best practice is the one you actually do.

Step 1: Clarify Your Sense of Purpose

The first step is to clarify what truly matters to you. There are many ways to practice this step. You can reflect on your life and note the causes you devote yourself to. Look for areas of interest. Maybe you like to help children or animals. Maybe you're passionate about the environment, get energized whenever the topic comes up in conversation, and read everything you can get your hands on. Or maybe you're always bringing people together at work and discover that part of your purpose is to create a sense of community.

Similarly, you can unearth your purpose by reflecting on a meaningful memory. When you think back to the moments of your life that were the most meaningful and fulfilling, what comes to mind? Once you remember something, dig a little deeper. What made this experience so meaningful? Why does it stand out? Let's say that you remember an important personal milestone like graduating from school. This may represent the power of perseverance and hard work or your belief in the importance of education. You might find many layers of purpose in a single memory. The key is to clarify the most uplifting and energizing ones for you now.

There are many ways to bring your purpose to the surface. Experiment and see what works best for you. This inner clarity is the foundation for a strong sense of purpose. It will give you a clear picture of what gives your life meaning.

Step 2: Apply Your Purpose in Daily Life

Once you've clarified an important purpose, the next step is to bring it into your daily life. When it comes to applying purpose to our everyday lives, we often think we need to completely change how we live and what we do. You might think you need to quit your job or spend more time volunteering for an important cause. Although doing meaningful things is indeed important, when it comes to the skill of purpose, it's more about shifting your perspective.

Start by recognizing the areas in your life where you already embody your purpose. For instance, if you value education, look for all the small things you already do that express your commitment to lifelong learning. Maybe you read books like this to keep broadening your perspective. Maybe you listen to podcasts to get new perspectives and learn about the world. Maybe you are naturally curious and love to hear about other people and learn about their lives. The key is to find this sense of purpose in the life you already lead and the things you already do. Acknowledge these moments and appreciate how they align with your sense of purpose. With this shift in perspective, you will see your life and pursuits through the lens of your purpose, which will allow you to bring meaning and fulfillment into the flow of your everyday life.

In addition to exploring all the areas where you already embody a sense of purpose, experiment with applying it in new situations. If you love art and want the world to be filled with creativity, for example, look for ways to express this in your relationships. Share an image of your favorite piece of art with someone you know who might appreciate it. Make a plan to visit a gallery or a museum once a week or to treat a friend to an interesting new movie. These may be things you already do, but if you do them consciously to align with a deeper sense of purpose, they will take on new meaning and depth.

Step 3: Extend Your Perspective to Mundane and Challenging Situations

With practice, you will get good at bringing your purpose to life in the more obvious areas, but there will likely be activities and routines that still seem meaningless. So the third step is to apply this new perspective to mundane and challenging situations. Begin by looking at routine tasks through the lens of your guiding purpose. How might tidying up your home be an expression of your purpose? How might getting your work done on time be linked to your purpose?

Eventually, you can experiment with applying this perspective to stressful situations. When faced with challenges, try to see them as opportunities to deepen your sense of purpose. For example, how might you see a difficult project at work or a tense argument with a partner or a friend as part of your purpose? See if you can reframe these situations as opportunities to express your deeper motivations, even when you feel threatened. With practice, you will learn to approach difficult situations with a broader perspective. You will naturally feel more confident, and difficult situations will reinforce your sense of purpose.

Developing a sense of purpose isn't about finding the perfect job or achieving some grand goal like ending world hunger. It's about cultivating a way of seeing the world that allows you to find meaning and fulfillment in everything you do. It's about weaving your core principles into the fabric of your everyday existence. With these three steps, you will gradually learn to find meaning in your life's highs and lows and everything in between. Remember, this is an ongoing process. Revisit your guiding purpose daily, tweak your perspective as needed, and navigate life's twists and turns with purpose as your compass.

REFLECTIVE WRITING PRACTICE

Reframe a Current Challenge

There are many ways to practice the skill of purpose, from meditative self-reflection to meaningful dialogue with a therapist, partner, or friend. Here, we will use journaling to reflect on a challenging situation and view it as an opportunity to cultivate a sense of purpose.

Before you begin journaling, pause and rest your mind for a few moments. Feel the movement of your breath. Allow your body and mind to relax and give yourself the space to simply be for a few moments.

When you feel ready, begin the reflection with pen and paper. Start by bringing to mind a difficult or stressful situation you are currently facing, but not one that feels too intense or overwhelming. It's important to start with one that feels workable.

What comes up when you bring this situation to mind? Write down the feelings, thoughts, memories, and expectations that arise in your mind. As you do this, feel free to pause from time to time to observe your inner experience with curiosity and warmth. Treat this as a light exercise. There's no right or wrong experience to have. Simply observe and note what you find.

Next, ask yourself, *How would I handle this situation when I'm at my very best? What would that look like? How would I see things?* Again, take a few moments to reflect on these questions and write down your thoughts or reflections.

Now, dig a little deeper. What is guiding you when you think about what it might look like to handle this situation well? Is there an important principle or a sense of purpose underneath? Maybe integrity or the belief that everyone deserves a second chance is a guiding principle. See if you can use the situation to clarify a deeper sense of purpose and write down the thoughts that come to mind.

For the final step, think about the coming days and weeks. When will you find yourself dealing with this situation? How might you use it as an opportunity to further this reflection and practice the skill of purpose? See if you can jot down some ideas and notes to guide yourself next time you deal with this difficult situation.

You can end as you began, with a few moments of restful awareness. Pause for a few moments. Take a few slow, deep breaths. Notice any thoughts and feelings that are present. Rest your mind for a few moments before you move on with your day.

Post-Traumatic Growth

Sometimes, we feel overwhelmed by life's struggles yet pull through somehow, as was the case with Nelson Mandela during his many years in prison. Sometimes, we even grow through adversity, taking important lessons into the rest of our lives. Research shows that when life's difficulties bring out the best in us, purpose can play a central role.

Scientists have shown that human beings respond to major traumas in a few different ways. On one end of the spectrum is post-traumatic stress disorder (PTSD), which develops when facing a major challenge knocks the nervous system out of balance. The challenge triggers a stress response that keeps playing out long after the situation has passed. On the other end of the spectrum is what scientists call post-traumatic growth, which occurs when a highly challenging life situation results in positive growth and transformation. People who experience post-traumatic growth often report finding more purpose in life. They focus their energy on things that truly matter—for instance, spending more time with loved ones. A study of nearly 4,000 US military veterans found that a sense of purpose is one of the factors linked to post-traumatic growth. Another study found that purpose in life can help us cope with something as devastating as an earthquake. In a group of 200 earthquake survivors in Pakistan, higher levels of purpose were linked to lower levels of PTSD symptoms and higher levels of positive emotions, which are associated with both physical and mental health.

Some of the most interesting science on this topic has focused on cancer patients. Scientists have observed that some cancer patients seem to undergo a profound personal transformation over the course of their illness. They begin to link the small details of life and routine interactions with other people to a deeper sense of purpose. The key to this transformation is often what scientists call reappraisal. The illness forces cancer patients to rethink their lives and priorities and reflect on what's truly important. And as a result, they discover a clarity of purpose they missed before their cancer diagnosis.

Every one of us will face a range of challenges in life. How can we prepare ourselves to meet them with grace? Or to bring a fresh perspective to the ones we've already faced? Purpose is the key. Clarity of purpose doesn't give us a life free from problems, but it does give us the tools and resources to weather life's storms. Purpose helps us stop avoiding or ignoring our problems with the hope that they'll just disappear. Instead, we learn to open to these struggles and see what they have to teach us. We find ways to learn, grow, and even imagine how we might use our struggles to benefit others.

Remember that this shift in perspective doesn't invalidate or minimize what we're going through. It certainly doesn't rationalize the injustice of the world or justify harmful behavior. What it does do is give us the inner resources to deal with adversity. It helps us focus on what we can influence and make peace with what we can't.

How to Build a Meaningful Life

It's natural for peak experiences and meaningful moments to come to mind when we think of our purpose. When aligned with our purpose, we have some of the most outstanding moments of our lives. But hopefully, it is now clear that the real skill is transforming our perspective so that our daily routines and activities, major life challenges, and unexpected changes are infused with this sense of purpose. An inspiring example of this comes from Viktor Frankl's *Man's Search for Meaning*. A Holocaust survivor, Frankl lost his parents, his brother, and his wife in the concentration camps. Only his sister, who had left Europe for Australia, survived. Frankl himself endured unimaginable suffering and witnessed horrific acts of cruelty during the war. He later wrote that meaning and purpose were the keys to his survival. Beyond his own experience, he wrote that the quest to find meaning in life is not only central to human flourishing but, perhaps more importantly, precisely what helps us endure life's most challenging moments. Frankl's aspiration to share this message with the world kept him going. He saw himself as part of something bigger and wanted to play a role in helping the world move in a better direction. He envisioned a day when people would understand the importance of finding meaning in life, even in the face of tremendous suffering.

No one would ever choose to undergo what Frankl experienced, but his example shows how a clear sense of purpose can help us see our lives from a new perspective. While it doesn't justify the harm done by others or the suffering that comes our way, a sense of purpose can help us keep our spirit alive as we reframe the adversity. Maybe our challenges help us better understand what others face and what we can do to help. Maybe our sadness and pain can be channeled into creative expression. Some of the most beautiful works of art are the product of deep suffering. We can discover a tremendous reservoir of inner strength and resilience in times of adversity. These are the moments when a sense of purpose can be a raft that helps us stay afloat in life's turbulent waters. In Frankl's case, his personal tragedy became the means through which he helped so many others.

It's clear that purpose is more than a philosophical idea. It's a profound force for well-being, supported by extensive scientific research. A clear sense of purpose can positively impact our physical health, resilience, and cognitive abilities. Purpose acts like a psychological immune system, strengthening us in times of stress and helping us recover from adversity. Whether it helps us view a stressful conversation as a chance to practice patience, see household tasks as a way to care for loved ones, or reframe work challenges as opportunities for growth, purpose gives us a new lens through which to view our everyday experiences. The beauty of purpose lies in its accessibility. We don't need to change our circumstances or achieve great things to live purposefully. We simply need to bring awareness to the meaning already present in our daily lives and let it guide us forward.

Part Three

Flourishing Every Day

Chapter 9

Making Flourishing a Habit

We are what we repeatedly do. Excellence, then, is not an act, but a habit.

—Aristotle

Richie leads what most others would consider a very stressful life. He works constantly. A recent audit of his calendar by one of his staff indicated that in a recent month, he had calendared an average of seventy-three working hours per week. It is not unusual for him to have twelve-hour workdays and then do at least another two hours of work in the evening. He typically travels at least twice per month. All of this adds up to a great deal of daily stress. When Richie is home, he adopts a routine to help him manage the crazy life he leads. He begins his days with a ritual of morning meditation, usually followed by a porridge breakfast (oatmeal with some added extras), with generous fruit and nut toppings. Susan, his wife, makes the porridge for him a few times a week so that all Richie has to do is heat it up in the morning while he boils water for Susan's tea. As he waits for the porridge and water to heat up, he reflects on the joy of breakfast and the day ahead. Another opportunity to help relieve suffering and promote more flourishing. Once he sits down to eat, he spends a minute in silence, reflecting on the many causes and conditions that come together to create this very wholesome breakfast. He thinks of his wife, who made the porridge, and then he thinks of the farmers who harvested the grains, fruits, and nuts, the people who made their dishes, the kitchen table, and everyone who transported and sold the food he is fortunate to eat. This moment of reflection kindles a deep sense of appreciation as it reveals the interdependence that's necessary for the everyday act of eating. Together these simple, small acts of appreciation and kindness are like elixirs for the soul and they help Richie achieve at least a modicum of balance in his life.

Cort has his own ways of infusing his routines with intention. When his never-ending to-do list starts to feel overwhelming, he hits pause and goes for a walk, even if it's just a short stroll between meetings. It's not just the physical movement that helps. When he goes for a walk he always begins by forming a positive motivation. He brings to mind how going for a walk is one way he cares for his body and how bringing awareness and purpose to the activity is also a way he cares for his mind. He also forms the wish that the benefits from this daily walk will ripple out to others and help them flourish as well. By the end of this short reflection, the simple act of going for a walk has become part of a larger current of wisdom and compassion in the world. The walk itself is a moving meditation for Cort. Even a few minutes of mindful movement can bring a much-needed mental reset into his day.

Think about the routines in your life. What do you do every day that could be transformed into a meaningful and fulfilling activity? It could be something you're passionate about or something that's part of your morning or nighttime routine. It could even be a boring chore. With a little intention, any moment of your life can be infused with awareness, connection, insight, and purpose. It just takes practice.

Flourishing is a lifelong journey. When it comes to cultivating well-being, one of the most common challenges people face is forming and maintaining healthy habits. We've all experienced this challenge with our diet or exercise or our intention to let go of an unhealthy impulse. Fortunately, modern science has uncovered some of the most effective ways to stick with the habits that are good for us, and we can apply what's been learned to building the habit of flourishing. Using the four skills we've explored in this book, you can create new routines, and it's far more achievable than you might think.

Conscious Habits

Habits are behaviors that occur automatically in a specific context or that are cued by a particular person or situation. The behavior typically occurs without much thought or awareness. For example, taking the same route home after work is an automatic habit. We know it's automatic by what happens on the rare occasions when we must deviate from the usual pattern. If you need to change your route to pick up some groceries, for instance, you may find yourself following your typical route when you suddenly realize you've made a mistake and need to change direction to get to the grocery store. A habit is automatic. We don't think about it. The cues that trigger a pattern are the factors that feed a habit—in this case, the time of day, leaving work, and driving home. In other words, cues are the circumstances that set the stage for a habit. Despite the important role they play, we rarely notice these cues.

The flourishing skills we've looked at in this book are most beneficial when they become *conscious habits*. The idea of a "conscious habit" may seem like an oxymoron since habits are supposed to operate automatically without conscious awareness. But in our approach to making flourishing a habit, what's automatic is the triggering context, or the cues.

For example, in Richie's morning routine, making tea is the cue that automatically elicits Richie's conscious habit of reflection. The making of the tea is what psychologists call an "affordance"; making tea automatically affords Richie an opportunity to reflect on the action. However, the action itself and, most importantly, the intention behind it, become conscious—unlike a typical habit where the action remains automatic and unconscious.

The conscious habits of flourishing are powerful because they provide benefits on many levels. You get not only the benefit of the activity you're engaged in but also the added benefits of strengthening one or more flourishing skills and building up a repertoire of healthy psychological qualities that will serve you in other areas of life. For example, if you link a simple daily activity like tidying up your home to awareness, you will still get the end result of a clean living space but also the added benefit of training your mind. You'll have strengthened your ability to notice your mental and emotional states in real time and your ability to consciously regulate them. If you notice a healthy stream of thoughts or an emotional reaction that feels fulfilling, you can savor it. If a stream of toxic thoughts sweeps through your mind, you can either bring your awareness to the inner experience until the thoughts run their course or redirect your mind to something more wholesome. Just a few moments of cultivating a conscious habit this way can activate a wide range of beneficial inner experiences, rippling through your nervous system and brain chemistry and supporting your ability to flourish.

The key is to use the things you already do and the life you already lead as opportunities to practice. Cort, for instance, had to build new conscious habits when his son, CJ, was born. Cort was living in Kathmandu then and was immersed in his meditation training. His days were spent translating ancient texts, meditating, doing yoga, and spending time in intensive retreat each year, meditating for more than twelve hours a day for months on end. When CJ was born, Cort's world turned upside down.

At first, he struggled to adjust. Finding even a few minutes to meditate undisturbed felt like a distant memory. But he soon realized that his new circumstances were an opportunity. Holding on to the past wasn't helping anything; instead, he could embrace the precious moments with his newborn son and use them to practice. With this new perspective, he began experimenting. One of his "daddy duties" was putting CJ down for naps, so he transformed this daily ritual into a practice of love. As he lay there with CJ drifting off to sleep beside him, Cort tapped into his love and affection for his son and nurtured it. Sometimes, he simply savored the warm glow of love that filled his heart. Other times, he would shower CJ with affection, imagining warm rays of love flowing out from his heart to CJ. And sometimes, he would extend this love to others, sending it out into the world with the wish that everyone everywhere feel safe, protected, and loved. This became one of the most important rituals in Cort's life, one that he continued for more than three years when they moved back to the US and CJ began preschool. Cort's son is now in his twenties, but Cort still remembers that daily nap ritual as one of the most meaningful memories from his son's childhood.

As you can see from Cort's experience, building conscious habits of flourishing can transform everyday activities into opportunities for exploration and self-discovery. The outer expression of what you are doing isn't so important—it's the inner process that really matters. You can change a light bulb while consciously filling your heart with kindness or relax into awareness while stuck in traffic. You can even transform stressful moments into springboards for compassion, self-reflection, and insight.

The leap from unconscious, automatic behaviors to conscious habits takes more than intellectual understanding. It takes an experiential approach. There are so many instances of people saying to themselves and others that they "know" meditating would benefit them, but they still can't get themselves to do it. We see this pattern with other health-related behavioral changes we "know" would be good for us—better diets, more physical exercise, not smoking, etc. But despite knowing what's good for us, we don't apply the effort to make the changes. What we need is learning acquired through practice. It is skill-based and represented in brain systems that are totally different from those that represent just acquiring information.

A habit ensures the regularity of a behavior. In this case, we're interested in behaviors that support our flourishing. When physical exercise becomes a habit, we don't deliberate about whether or not to do it, we simply do it—and our health improves. No cognitive effort is required, and no real choice needs to happen. The behavior occurs automatically. Our hope is that cultivating the skills of flourishing will become a habit for you.

Inspiration, Intention, Action, and Repetition

To make flourishing a habit, let's break down the steps involved in the learning: inspiration, intention, action, and repetition. We use these four steps in a model that depends on both declarative and procedural learning. You'll see that some of the steps engage one or the other form of learning more strongly.

Inspiration

Inspiration is a critical first step in forming any new habit. If we want to flourish, we need to feel inspired to do so. The inspiration might come from admiring someone and wanting some of their secret sauce.

If they have a practice that nurtures their flourishing, it inspires us to do likewise.

For example, the Dalai Lama is a major inspiration for both of us. What is the Dalai Lama's secret sauce? Well, he practices all four flourishing skills. As we mentioned in the chapter on connection, he engages in various forms of meditation and other contemplative practices for four to five hours each day. This has been his discipline for more than seven decades. And it shows! Although most people wouldn't engage in such intensive practice, the Dalai Lama is an outlier who inspires a vision of what is possible. We often reflect on the Dalai Lama's dedication. If he can practice four to five hours a day well into his eighties, certainly we can practice for at least forty-five minutes a day.

But inspiration alone is not enough. Many of us have stories about being inspired by someone and setting the intention to make a practice more habitual only to find it difficult to sustain. Sometimes, our role model's way of doing things is beyond our reach. The Dalai Lama's daily practice is not something we strive to emulate because it isn't possible to practice four to five hours a day in the lives we lead. Although the mere fact of the Dalai Lama's extraordinary commitment to practice is a powerful statement, an inspiration won't be helpful if we use the person as a measuring stick. Instead, they give us direction, showing us what's possible and how we can move forward with a new sense of possibility and potential.

Sometimes, we may be inspired by someone who is radiant without knowing in detail what they might be doing to cultivate that radiance. Often, these are people who have faced significant hardships and been resilient in the face of adversity. They are kindhearted, generous people who exemplify the goodness that comes with connection, the second skill of flourishing. Just hearing their story can inspire a new habit.

Trevor Noah is one such person who radiates a warm heart and good nature. Although Trevor's childhood in apartheid South Africa was filled with trauma and violence, his loving mother helped to nurture his basic goodness. The trauma that was part of his upbringing probably played an important role in nurturing his empathy. Born in the ghetto of Johannesburg, Trevor's father was white and his mother Black. Interracial relationships and marriages were illegal when Trevor was born, so he had to spend a great deal of his childhood in hiding. He not only survived a very challenging early childhood under apartheid but also transformed his trauma through humor and went on to become a famous comedian. He has since created a foundation to help the youth in his native South Africa access quality education.

Of course, you don't have to be famous to follow your heart and engage in extraordinary acts of generosity. Everyday people can be just as inspiring on the path to flourishing. You don't have to look far. Consider the fact that every year more than 150 people in the United States donate a kidney to an unrelated, unknown individual. Such acts of altruism can inspire us to further develop our skills of connection and compassion and make flourishing a habit.

Intention

Intention is the purposeful, conscious decision or mental commitment to act, think, or behave in a certain way. Unlike accidental or spontaneous actions, intentions are deliberate and often reflect a person's deeper motivations and aspirations. For the skills of flourishing, setting a proper intention is the spark plug that ignites the process. According to the classic view of habit formation, once habits become fully established and automatic, intention is not required. For example, brushing our teeth is a daily habit we typically perform without intention. We don't consciously form an intention to brush our teeth. The very notion of automatic is the absence of conscious intention.

A conscious habit is very different. Conscious habits require intention—and intention will go a long way when bringing the four skills into your life. Forming an intention depends upon conscious awareness, though it can become automatic in response to a cue. Remember Richie's breakfast ritual? We can say that the presence of his wife's teacup is an affordance for the intentional appreciation practice Richie does when making tea and preparing breakfast. And remember Cort's daily strolls? Stepping out to go for a walk is another cue. It automatically gives rise to Cort's conscious intention to exercise for his benefit and the positive impact it can have on others.

Let's return to the habit of brushing your teeth. This is an automatic habit that you can transform into a conscious habit by piggybacking a flourishing skill onto it. In other words, brushing your teeth can become an affordance that automatically triggers a conscious intention. Maybe you want to set an intention to be aware of how the toothbrush feels on your teeth (awareness), or you could set an intention to reflect on people close to you and appreciate their positive qualities (connection). Maybe you want to set an intention to reflect on your current mental and emotional state and consider how your thoughts and feelings are shaping how you currently see yourself and the world (insight). Or your intention might be to reflect on how keeping your teeth and gums healthy is part of a general health routine that benefits you and your family since taking care of your health is also a way of taking care of them (purpose). Bringing intention to our automatic habits is a great way to practice all four skills of flourishing.

Action

Intention leads to action, the actual carrying out of a habit. The action can be physical or mental. For example, intentionally being aware or grateful are forms of mental action, while explicitly thanking someone or commending them are forms of physical action and expressions of the skill of connection. Whether the action is physical or mental, it arises from a conscious intention, and the process of engaging in the action helps form the habit of flourishing.

Cort and his wife, Kasumi, practice gratitude as part of their nighttime ritual. It always starts with a shared intention to transform the unconscious bedtime routine into a conscious practice. With this intention, they pick a person, situation, or memory and then take turns sharing three things they appreciate. In this practice, lying down in bed is the cue.

Similarly, when Richie greets a person, especially someone he's never met before, it's a cue for connection. For Richie, connecting involves directly looking into the other person's eyes, followed by a handshake and a genuine smile. These actions typically occur together, and they give Richie the experience of a meaningful exchange. The well-known philosopher Martin Buber referred to such moments of deep connection as an "I-Thou" experience, and it's more accessible than most of us believe. When Richie greets someone, his gaze and handshake are physical actions that help consolidate the psychological experience of connection.

This framework—moving from inspiration to intention to action—can help you benefit from the countless activities and routines in your daily life by transforming them into conscious habits. Take a moment to reflect on the flow of a typical day in your life. What's the first thing you do when you wake up in the morning? Imagine what the first few moments of each day might feel like if you spent those moments in mindful awareness, centering yourself before you begin your day. What if they were moments of inspiration and purpose, opportunities to infuse your day with direction and purpose? It takes only a few seconds to shift your perspective. The only thing you're adding to what you already do is intention. As you experiment with transforming routine activities into rituals, notice the specific actions you take. It may be the simple action of sitting down and placing food on the table. See if you can sense the feedback loop between intention and action and how they can reinforce each other to contribute to an elevated state of flourishing.

Repetition

Inspiration, intention, and action are essential, but repetition is the real key to habit formation. As we noted earlier, the science shows that different habits require different lengths of repetition to be established. Different lengths of time might also be required for different people. Still, repetition and practice are key in forming the habits for flourishing.

In 1999, *The New Yorker* published an article by Malcolm Gladwell on what makes people great at what they do. The article featured three people: the amazing hockey player Wayne Gretzky, the renowned cellist Yo-Yo Ma, and the accomplished neurosurgeon Charlie Wilson. Gladwell investigated what these three people had in common at the pinnacle of their professions. What he concluded was simple and profound: practice, practice, practice. These experts did not rely on already well-honed skills but continued to practice.

Practice and repetition are essential for forming a conscious habit. At the Center for Healthy Minds, we've discovered that repetition is more important than overall duration, particularly in the early stages of establishing a habit. Practicing for five minutes a day for thirty days is of greater benefit than practicing for thirty minutes on five different days of a month. Repetition is key.

Choose a flourishing habit you want to establish. You might want to reflect on your sense of purpose before you begin work each day or appreciate something about your partner whenever you see them. Maybe you want to wake up every morning and reflect on the preciousness of human life. Whatever habit you are trying to form, repetition is essential. Try keeping a calendar to track your efforts. At the end of each day, note whether you practiced the habit at least once that day, and see how many consecutive days you can repeat this habit. After about thirty days, notice whether the habit has become more regular or automatic.

Zeitgebers, Natural Time Cues

A zeitgeber is something that naturally occurs in the environment and provides a time cue. The word *zeitgeber* comes from the German *zeit*, meaning "time," and *geber*, or "giver." In science, we call the zeitgeber a "circadian time cue" because it is something that happens in sync with our biological rhythms. For example, the sun's rising and setting in the day-to-night cycle is a zeitgeber that tells you it's time to wake or sleep. Social zeitgebers are human-created events that mark time. For example, eating is a social zeitgeber; it's something humans do daily, often with other humans. Brushing our teeth in the morning is another social zeitgeber; it occurs daily and marks roughly the same time each day and night. Like cues, zeitgebers are powerful opportunities for habit formation.

We can easily add a conscious habit to a zeitgeber so that we remember to build it daily. Let's consider how we can use eating to support a habit of flourishing. The act of sitting down to eat can be a cue that automatically activates our conscious intention to do a short connection practice. The next time you sit down to eat, try the following practice, which you can do with your eyes open or closed.

Bring to mind some of the people who were involved in the

conditions that brought you this meal. It might be the person who cooked the food, the farmers who grew the vegetables, the truck driver who transported the food from farm to market, the grocery store staff, the person who helped you pick out your dishes, or the nephew who worked with you to fix the broken chair. Bring one of these people into your mind and heart, and allow your appreciation to arise. It doesn't matter whether you know the person. Reflect on the extraordinary web of connection that's needed to accomplish something as simple as sitting down to eat.

If you'd like, bring a second person into your mind and heart and repeat this reflection.

You don't need to spend more than a minute doing this. Whenever practical (perhaps for your meals at home), see if you can weave this connection practice into your mealtime and notice how it impacts your experience.

This eating practice is just one example of how you can build one of the skills for flourishing into your day. You might use the moment of the sun going down for an insight practice or your morning tea or coffee for a purpose practice. Whatever you choose, a true zeitgeber is something that occurs daily on a regular schedule. We don't need to remember to eat, brush our teeth, or have our morning beverage. Once you learn to make the association with your habit, the zeitgeber itself will automatically activate your conscious intention to engage in a short flourishing practice. We often call these short practices micro-supports. If you can sprinkle several micro-supports into your day, over time these practices can change your life.

Turning Poison into Medicine

Look around, and you'll find cues to build habits for flourishing everywhere, even in your challenges.

Earlier in their relationship, Cort and his wife often argued over little things. At a certain point, Cort realized the arguments weren't really about whatever sparked the disagreement. They were about the discomfort of feeling criticized and disappointing or upsetting his wife. Once he saw the pattern, he started to see these moments of tension as an opportunity. At first, his intention was to bring awareness to the situation, to notice his bodily reactions, the reactive thoughts spinning through his mind, and his impulse to defend himself. This completely dissolved the emotional pattern and opened up space for a different response. Now, the same moments that used to create tension are openings to reconnection and genuine conversation.

We all make mistakes. We all meet challenges. Opportunities to build new habits abound. Let's look at one more example since we're faced with challenges almost every day.

Think of a time when you were irritated with someone you work with. (Although we both wish we never got annoyed at work, we do. It happens to all of us.) Consider a time when someone you work with did not do what you wanted. Recall the wave of irritation that washed over you. The next time a situation like this happens, the moment you sense the irritation, allow it to become a cue to nurture compassion. Very often, the person upsetting us is trying their best but missing the mark for a good reason. It might be that they don't have all the information they need, are new to a task, or are stressed at home and didn't get enough sleep. As part of your compassion practice, you can reflect on such possibilities. This is a more compassionate view. For icing on the cake, you'll often find that the compassion you offer, even in heart and mind alone, is reciprocated. Warm exchanges like this can dramatically transform the workplace and help nurture collective well-being.

Establishing Your Flourishing Habits

When Richie's son went on his first meditation retreat, he asked the teacher how to establish a daily meditation practice. "Just touch your meditation cushion every day, even if you can't practice," the teacher told him. This wise guidance helped Richie's son use his meditation cushion, a powerful symbol for the practice, not to meditate so much as to remind him to practice informally throughout his day.

While establishing a new habit is never easy, it's often easier than you think, especially for habits of flourishing. You don't need to meditate for long periods; you simply need to use your mind intentionally. Sprinkling moments of recognition and reflection into your daily life will add up, and they can lead to shifts in your flourishing. Forming habits can be challenging for all of us, and even once a habit is fully established, it might still require effort. But with time, practice, and approaches like the ones we've suggested in this chapter and throughout the book, new habits will unfold more easily. One day, you will find yourself practicing the skills of flourishing without having to decide whether you should. It will simply happen. And when these habits begin to happen spontaneously, you will begin to taste the sweetness of flourishing!

Chapter 10

Change Your Mind, Change the World

Progress is impossible without change, and those who cannot change their minds cannot change anything.

—George Bernard Shaw

By now, we hope you're feeling optimistic about the flourishing that is possible in your life. You've learned about neuroplasticity, epigenetics, and the basic machinery of your brain and body, which is more pliable than you might have imagined. You really can change. Our minds are not fixed. Our capacity to flourish has been there from the beginning. We all have what it takes. We simply need to recognize this truth and nurture the capacities we carry within.

The problems facing our world today are largely of our own making. Our world is filled with divisiveness and political polarization, loneliness and depression, distractibility that is off the charts, and decision-making that prioritizes immediate gains over long-term outcomes that would serve the greater good. These are all symptoms of a deeper problem that reflects an untapped potential to flourish.

As you've learned, intentionally using your mind for a few minutes each day to nurture the skills of flourishing can make an enormous difference. In light of the perfect storm of challenges before us, let's all commit to spreading the message that we are born to flourish and that it can be learned. When enough of us nurture these qualities, our communities will become healthier, and a collective field of flourishing can arise to further support our individual efforts.

The two of us, Richie and Cort, frequently hear the concern that helping people in unjust systems or organizations improve their well-being could pacify them and detract from the need to change these systems and organizations. We are sensitive to this concern. While there are organizations and systems so corrupt and toxic that the best strategy is to leave them if possible, we also know that individual change and systemic change go hand in hand. Organizations are made up of people, and if we want an organization to change, the people in it need to change. What's more, burnout is all too common among change agents and social activists. Flourishing will strengthen their vitality and resilience, making them better and more effective and reducing the likelihood of burnout.

As we're increasingly called upon to recognize how our individual and collective flourishing are intimately linked, let's not forget our relationship to the land, to nature, to Mother Earth. We sometimes forget about this connection, but recent fires, hurricanes, and earthquakes are dramatic reminders of our intimate connection with the natural world.

Anger and despair are very understandable given the state of the world. Still, they only make us miserable and undermine the very inner resources that give us the strength to address the monumental problems we face as a species. Training ourselves to flourish by practicing the skills we've explored in this book presents a different way to live. Instead of feeling overwhelmed and powerless, we can tap into innate capacities we all have yet rarely recognize. These qualities are within each of us, and nurturing them anchors us to a way of being that is life-affirming and empowering. As we begin to tap our full potential to live with more awareness, connection, insight, and purpose, we will naturally feel more capable of managing the ups and downs of our own lives, and perhaps even see our personal journeys as part of something much bigger.

To Flourish Is to Energize

Ronan Harrington was a leader of the Extinction Rebellion in the UK, an environmental movement dedicated to taking action on the climate crisis. Ronan was on the barricades, playing a key leadership role in this organization, but after years of pushing himself for the cause, he completely burned out. He suffered from debilitating chronic pain and attributed this, in large part, to his role in Extinction Rebellion.

Ronan had an epiphany in a meeting with the Dalai Lama. This was a two-day meeting in Dharamsala where fifteen young leaders were each given about ten minutes to share their story, followed by some discussion. At the end of the first day, Ronan challenged the Dalai Lama. We had never heard anyone speak as forcefully to the Dalai Lama as Ronan did that day. Ronan told the Dalai Lama that all the discussion about common humanity was just talk and accused him of using empty platitudes. The Dalai Lama's response was gentle. He repeated what he'd previously explained, that change needs to begin within and that our authentic transformation together will only occur in this way.

In between our meetings with the Dalai Lama, we met as a group to process all that was occurring. We had the benefit of two Tibetan meditation masters, Tsoknyi Rinpoche and Yongey Mingyur Rinpoche (who happened to be brothers), teaching us meditation to cultivate awareness, connection, and insight. Ronan was beginning to taste the possibility of living a different way without abandoning his commitment to activism. When we all met again with the Dalai Lama the following morning, something had shifted in Ronan. His perspective had begun to widen as he began to envision the possibility of truly embodying peace.

This wake-up call in Dharamsala profoundly impacted Ronan's life and career. While his chronic pain did not subside at first, his relationship to the pain began to change. He no longer defined himself as "being in pain." Gradually, the pain subsided, and Ronan was able to live a more balanced life. He recognized that he could use his experience as an example to help nurture balance and resilience in others. Ronan is now a sought-after consultant and speaker on the global stage who shares his inspiring story to help others in high-pressure situations discover the vitality they also carry within.

Ever-Widening Circles

When individuals in a community flourish, the entire community is more likely to flourish. We saw this in our work with the school system in Louisville, Kentucky, where we trained teachers and administrative staff in the four skills of flourishing. As their well-being improved, everyone's perception of the organization shifted. The administration reported a decrease in anxiety, depression, and stress and an increase in their ability to flourish, while the teachers reported a marked difference in their perception of the administrative staff. Cultivating the four skills of flourishing heightened everyone's appreciation of and trust in one another, and these changes became stronger over time. In the five-month follow-up, they were more pronounced. In short, as everyone on staff practiced the flourishing skills we taught them, they demonstrated the power of a collective to transform an organization for the better. The employees of the Louisville school system became more welcoming, enjoyed a greater sense of belonging, and felt a stronger sense of purpose.

Several years ago, Richie had the opportunity to visit an elementary school in Israel in an impoverished area of south Tel Aviv. Tel Hai was an integrated Arab and Jewish school with a lot of violence and a poor academic record. Nava Levit-Binnun, a dear friend and professor at the Reichman University in Herzliya, Israel, and her colleague Nimrod Sheinman worked with this school for five years, bringing simple flourishing practices to the staff, students, and the students' parents. They were invited to do so by the school's principal, who was frightened by the violence and concerned about students' poor academic outcomes.

Although the intervention was not explicitly based on our flourishing framework (it had yet to be published), theirs did focus on two of the skills of flourishing, awareness and connection. The intervention dramatically transformed the school's culture. Strengthening everyone's skills of awareness and connection alone reduced the violence. Even the neighborhood around the school was positively impacted. The school's academic performance shifted, too. Before the introduction of the flourishing curriculum (a one-hour weekly class), students were chronically underachieving, but five years after the curriculum's introduction, students scored higher than the national average on Israel's standardized tests, known as GEMS, Growth and Effectiveness Measures for Schools. What began as a simple intervention targeting staff, students, and students' parents morphed into a system-wide transformation.

Improving academic performance was not a goal of this intervention. It was implemented to help stem the tide of violence and improve the students' socio-emotional outcomes. The improvement in academic performance is similar to the outcomes we saw in

Louisville, Kentucky. When teachers are more present and connected with students, and students are more present, relaxed, and connected to their teachers, peers, and parents, the students learn better. When their minds are less cluttered with anxious and depressing thoughts, they can more effectively focus on the learning task at hand.

During the fourth year of this program at the Tel Hai school, Richie met with the school's principal, who told him the skills she learned had renewed her vitality and sense of purpose. She explained that her first year at the school had been tremendously difficult. The violence was so terrifying she requested an unpaid leave of absence her second year. During this time, she discovered contemplative-based approaches to flourishing and became determined to bring these practices to the school. She met Nava and Nimrod, and together they embarked upon this remarkable program when she returned to her job the following year.

Are you part of a group or organization that is dysfunctional in some way? Would a flourishing intervention that reaches most, if not all, of the group's members be possible? Can you envision a different operating system for the organization? How can you apply the inspiration these schools offer to the group you're a part of?

The Need for Purpose

While purpose is a core characteristic of flourishing for teens, it is likely the most important flourishing skill for older adults. We know that having a strong sense of purpose is the most important psychological predictor of longevity among people 70 years of age and older.

At the time of this book's writing, about 17 percent of the US population is 65 years or older, and this percentage is expected to increase to at least 22 percent by 2040. As the aging population increases, life expectancy is also increasing. The average life expectancy in the US at the time of this writing is about 77 years; among women, it is higher—more than 80 years. After the kids have grown and after retirement, many older adults struggle with a sense of purpose in their lives, and purpose, as we've seen, is central to our ability to flourish. For this reason, practicing the fourth skill of flourishing can be especially beneficial to those in their later years.

About twenty years ago, a group at Johns Hopkins University birthed a brilliant project in Baltimore, Maryland, designed to give retired persons (mostly women) an opportunity to connect to their sense of purpose by helping neighborhood youth. Experience Corps is a program that recruits women between the ages of 60 and 86 to volunteer as aides in the local public elementary schools. In the original program, 95 percent of the volunteers were low-income African Americans. Eighty-two percent had no education beyond high school, and 70 percent had an average income below $15,000 a year. The women were each asked to volunteer 15 hours a week. Before beginning their volunteer work, they received 30 hours of training across two weeks.

The presence of these elders in the elementary schools was a godsend! They helped in the cafeteria during lunch hour, showed kids how to use the library and select appropriate books, read to the children, and during playtime helped the children resolve conflict in an emotionally intelligent way. What was remarkable about this program was that it produced strong benefits for both the elders and the kids.

Research by the Johns Hopkins group shows that these elders had significant improvements in their cognitive and emotional skills as well as their physical conditioning. They showed improvements in walking speed compared to a control group, and they showed improvements in executive function (the capacity to direct their attention and regulate their behavior). MRI scans on a subset of these individuals showed functional brain changes. The activity of the prefrontal cortex, a key node in the central executive system, increased, which was associated with increases in executive function. Most importantly, these women showed a renewed sense of purpose, and it's likely that many, if not most, of the other benefits they enjoyed flowed from their renewed sense of purpose.

The results from Experience Corps are inspiring. Giving seniors the opportunity to volunteer and help kids in their neighborhood dramatically elevated their sense of purpose and greatly benefited both the kids and themselves. This program is now being scaled throughout the United States by AARP, which has taken it over. In 2023, Experience Corps was operating in twenty communities and involved more than 1,000 senior volunteers. Imagine if something like Experience Corps were introduced in other sectors—for example, in health care. Senior volunteers might assist in hospital settings and benefit both themselves and the patients they serve. Making simple acts of altruism more readily available has multiplicative benefits!

Remembering and Forgetting

We've provided the ingredients necessary to flourish. But each of us needs to discover our own best recipe. No single formula is right for everyone. What is important, however, is that you take time to practice all four of the skills. Establish daily rituals that you can commit to, and use the habit-forming tips we shared in chapter 9 to integrate habits of flourishing into your daily life. Organize your daily life and social events around awareness, connection, insight, and purpose. If you look closely, you'll discover that your life is filled with opportunities to practice.

It can be easy to forget the habits of flourishing when life gets overwhelming, when the people we love are suffering, when we're in the thick of our daily lives. We all get knocked off track. Although we promised ourselves we'd practice every day, we might sit down and mindlessly take the first bite of food at our meal without expressing appreciation for the many people it took to bring our food to the table or begin a workday without reflecting on the purpose of our work. At times, we can also be so focused on our next activity that we forget to bring awareness to the present moment and pay little attention to the feelings and sensations in our bodies now.

It's okay. Even with more than sixty years of cumulative meditation experience between the two of us, we, too, forget to apply what we know will be helpful in a messy situation. So, how can we remind ourselves to use our minds intentionally?

Sometimes, a reminder can be a quote or a picture of someone or someplace you love and admire. It might be a song you wake up to in the morning. It could be a symbolic object, something someone gave you that has personal significance. These little objects we arrange in our homes, cars, and workplaces can support us in the heat of the moment or when we forget to practice. And if we get used to these reminders and they lose their impact, we can switch them up to keep them fresh.

Richie has a picture of his meditation teacher on his Apple Watch as a continuous reminder throughout the day. The desk in the study of his home is replete with reminders. He keeps photos of teachers who have inspired him, quotes that open his mind, and pictures of loved ones who keep him connected to his heart. In every direction Richie turns, there are reminders. About every six months, he rotates or replaces them with something else. Little touchpoints like these sprinkled into everyday life help make flourishing real by reminding us to use our minds intentionally and not to squander our opportunities.

Building Flourishing Cities

At the Center for Healthy Minds, we have a dream of flourishing cities. Imagine a city of moderate size, say about one million people, in which most people embrace the possibility of flourishing as a quality that can be nurtured. Billboards and ads on city transportation could relay reminders with this message. Public service announcements on local television and radio would provide resources to help citizens develop the four skills of flourishing. City government, health care, education, first responders, communities of faith, businesses and workplaces, all these major sectors of the city would be on board. The digital platforms they use—for example, electronic medical records in health care—would be designed to include simple micro-supports with in-the-moment practices to help patients, clients, and colleagues better interact. Imagine a city mayor championing the work and the possibility of this city as a model for the world. If everyone in the city nurtured their flourishing for even a few minutes a day, the city would inevitably be transformed. Flourishing would be the talk of the town!

How might we document the benefits of this radical experiment? We would look for distal outcomes that matter. Distal outcomes that matter are those real-life outcomes that all societies care about, such as the city's crime rate, suicide rate, addiction rate, life expectancy, and health care costs. We already know that training the mind to flourish affects our biology and health: inflammatory molecules are down-regulated, stress biology is transformed, and brain health is improved. Health impacts would be even easier to discern when training to flourish is scaled. We would expect to see health, health care, and health care costs improve. We would also expect people to live longer. Training educators in the four flourishing skills has also already demonstrated a positive trickle-down effect that benefits students. So we could expect school attendance, standardized test scores, and high school graduation rates to improve. Of course, we would have economists track the savings that would accrue from all these outcomes. And if we find what we expect, this would truly be a game changer, with other cities clamoring to adopt this approach.

We still have a long way to go before such a project is embraced. But as we document in this book, real progress is being made, and the evidence that training the mind can change the world is expanding exponentially.

Sharing with Others, Building the Movement

The most effective advertisement for the benefits of the approach to flourishing we offer in this book is for you to embody the qualities described—to show up fully present and aware, connected, self-reflective, and with purpose. When we walk the talk, we radiate these qualities, and others will notice. The power of community can be experienced through this kind of osmosis in social learning.

We are living in very challenging and complex times. The future of humanity demands we recalibrate. Remember: you were born with the capacity to flourish. We come into the world with the potential. What we each need to do is nurture it by practicing the skills that optimize our capacities. The evidence shows that it doesn't take much. If each of us spent as little time nourishing our minds daily as we do brushing our teeth, this world would really be so much more benevolent.

Please join us on this journey. There was never a time in human history when this message was more important than it is today. The future of humanity is at stake. And what is remarkable is that training the skills of our own flourishing benefits the greater good and vice versa. It is a virtuous cycle.

Acknowledgments

This book is the result of a lifelong journey of exploration and inquiry. We are profoundly grateful to the many teachers, colleagues, and loved ones who have shaped and supported us along the way.

First and foremost, we offer our deepest gratitude to our spiritual teachers, whose wisdom and compassion continue to inspire and guide our work. His Holiness the Dalai Lama has been a source of unending encouragement, reminding us time and again that human flourishing is not just possible but essential. We are especially grateful to our teacher, Yongey Mingyur Rinpoche, whose profound teachings have illuminated the path for us and so many others. His dedication to bridging ancient wisdom with modern science has been a guiding light for this work.

We are also indebted to our scientific colleagues and collaborators, particularly those at the Center for Healthy Minds at the University of Wisconsin–Madison. The research presented in this book builds on the collective efforts of an extraordinary community of scientists, researchers, and practitioners who have devoted their lives to understanding the nature of human flourishing. In particular, we wish to thank Christy Wilson-Mendenhall, whose insights and partnership in coauthoring our paper on the Healthy Minds Framework helped lay the scientific foundation for many of the ideas in this book, along with Simon Goldberg and Matt Hirshberg, who have been pioneers in the empirical research with the Healthy Minds Program.

Richie also thanks Dalal Abu Amneh, a recent visitor to our Center from Palestine, who has broadened his understanding of contemplative practice and contemplative science.

The work of Humin (formerly Healthy Minds Innovations) has played a critical role in translating research into accessible, practical tools for cultivating well-being. We are grateful to our colleagues there for their tireless efforts in developing the Healthy Minds Program (available as a mobile application and also taught in other formats) and so many other tools to bring our insights to life so they can touch the lives of countless people around the world. We are especially grateful to our CEO, Christina Glavas, and our chief science officer and COO, Raquel Tatar. We are also so thankful for the tireless advice and support of Steve Arnold, our longtime chair of the Humin board of directors.

A special thank-you to our friends and colleagues at Tergar International and the Tergar meditation community, whose dedication to deep practice and making these teachings widely available continues to inspire us. This global community of practitioners is living proof that flourishing is not a distant ideal but an ever-present possibility in our daily lives.

Books are not written in isolation, and this one has benefited from the insights, editorial guidance, and encouragement of many individuals. We would especially like to thank Haven Iverson, who helped us find our shared voice and carefully edited the raw materials of our original writings into something far more polished, as well as Vesela Simic, who brought great care and insight to another round of editing. Our work was also guided by Caroline Sutton, our editor at Avid Reader Press, who provided invaluable feedback that helped shape and refine our message, and our literary agent, Linda Loewenthal, who believed in the importance of this project from the beginning and shepherded the writing of this book from the moment it was an unformed idea in our heads to the final publication.

Our deepest gratitude goes to our families, whose love and support make everything possible. Richie wishes to thank his wife, Susan, for her unwavering support and wisdom throughout their journey together, and his children, Amelie and Seth, and grandkids, Soli, Aviva, Louie, and Sklar, who continue to be his greatest teachers. Cort expresses profound gratitude to his wife, Kasumi, whose patience, encouragement, and insight have been essential to his work and writing, and to his son, CJ, who has taught him more about flourishing than any scientific study could.

Finally, we acknowledge the countless research participants, students, and individuals around the world who have shared their experiences with us and participated in our studies. Your willingness to explore your minds and share your insights has advanced our understanding of human flourishing in ways that would otherwise be impossible. This book belongs to all of you as much as it does to us.

With a deep bow of gratitude,

Richie and Cort

Appendix

Additional Practices for Cultivating the Four Skills

In each of the skills chapters, we offered you a taste of the skill and a few ways to make that skill a part of your everyday life. But there are many ways to practice the four skills we've presented in these pages. This appendix contains simple instructions for four of the most widely practiced methods: sitting meditation, active meditation, journaling, and interpersonal practices. A few we have already mentioned; others are new. We encourage you to experiment with all four and focus on the forms of practice that best fit your interests and circumstances. The important thing is to make sure you take a few minutes to practice all four of the skills each and every day for flourishing to take off.

The Healthy Minds Meditation

Our first practice will combine elements of all four skills. If you only have time for one practice a day, we recommend this one. You can practice at any time of day, even during a short timeout at work.

Begin your meditation by reflecting on your motivation to practice. Link your meditation to a sense of purpose by imagining that what you are doing is part of a much larger current in the world. By doing this practice right now, you are doing your part to bring more awareness, connection, insight, and purpose into the world.

Once you feel connected to a sense of purpose, observe whatever happens in your mind. You don't need to focus or concentrate. Instead, let go and rest as you gently observe all the thoughts, feelings, impressions, and impulses that pass through your mind.

Next, bring in a spark of insight by exploring how rich and complex your experience is. To do this, you can start by giving a label to your current mental and emotional state, something like "tired," "relaxed," or "restless." Next, look beneath the label. What does that label actually refer to in your direct experience? Step back and observe what is happening in your body and mind and notice the many elements of your inner experience that you lump together and label.

After examining your inner experience, you can again let go and simply be present. Observe everything happening in your body and mind without judgment, just a light touch of warmth, openness, and curiosity.

To conclude the meditation, think about ways you can bring more presence, wisdom, and compassion into your interactions and relationships with others. Who will you see or interact with next? As you transition out of the practice, see if you can carry your meditation into these relationships.

Appendix

Additional Practices for the Skill of Awareness

AWARENESS PRACTICE #1

Sitting Meditation — Breathing with Awareness

Bring awareness to your posture as you find a comfortable, balanced position. Feel free to keep your eyes gently closed or open in a relaxed gaze if you find that more comfortable. Find a position that helps you feel wakeful and alert while also calm and relaxed. As you settle into a balanced posture, bring awareness to your body and notice how you feel.

Next, form an uplifting motivation by linking your practice to the greater good. Imagine how the positive effects of this practice might ripple out and bring more awareness, compassion, and wisdom into the world.

Now, take a few moments to shift from doing to a state of simply being. Give yourself some space to exist, without needing to do or change anything.

Gently bring your awareness to your breath. Take three slow, calming breaths and allow your body and mind to relax with each exhalation.

After three deep breaths, let your breath return to its normal pace and begin to count your breath. Breathe in and out, and then count "1" in your mind after the exhalation, then "2" for the next cycle of breathing. Go up to 3 cycles of breathing and then begin again at 1.

When you get distracted, which may happen many times in a meditation session, simply notice this and appreciate that you have noticed the pull of distraction. Then bring your attention back to your breath and begin again at 1.

Continue counting your breath for 5, 10, or even 20 minutes, depending on how long your session is.

If your mind grows more calm and settled, you can move on to the second step of breath awareness practice: feeling the breath. Let go of the counting and notice where you feel the movement of your breath most clearly. It may be in your nostrils or at the tip of your nose, at the base of your throat, your sternum, or your navel area.

Gently rest your awareness in this part of your body. At the same time, allow your awareness to spread throughout your entire body, as though you can feel your entire body breathing, with the center in your area of focus.

Feel the nourishing, energizing quality of your breath. Feel its healing energy spread through your body.

You can continue this part of the practice as long as you like, from a few minutes up to 10 or 20 minutes if you have time.

When your mind grows even more calm and stable, you can add a third step: being with the breath. At this stage, you can let the field of your attention be wide and expansive. Feel your entire body breathing with a very light, almost effortless, touch of awareness. If you know you are breathing, that's enough. There is no focus or mental effort required at this stage.

As before, when you notice the pull of distraction, celebrate that moment of noticing the old habit of the wandering mind, bring yourself back to your breath, and begin again.

Appendix

You can conclude your practice by releasing your focus on your breath and just sit for a few moments without any effort to adjust or control your attention.

As you transition out of the meditation, bring awareness into whatever you do next in your day. Use every activity and interaction as an opportunity to practice the skill of awareness.

AWARENESS PRACTICE #2

Active Meditation — Morning Routine with Awareness

Active meditations use the natural rhythms of everyday activities as supports for practice. For this particular practice, use your normal morning routine as a period of formal meditation practice. Set a timer for a particular period, from 5 to 20 minutes, and set a clear intention to be mindful and aware of whatever you do in this period. You can use whatever activities you do, like listening to a podcast or music or sending and receiving messages as the basis for your practice.

Bring your full attention to the sensory experience of what you are doing. If you are in the bathroom brushing your teeth, for example, attend to the physical sensations of brushing and the sound of water. If you are in the kitchen, notice all the sounds around you and everything you see and hear. As you practice, your mind will naturally think of other things, pulling you out of the present moment and into the past or future. Simply notice this when it happens without judgment and celebrate the fact that you are noticing moments of distraction. The more moments you notice, the more you will strengthen the brain networks that support your ability to be calm and focused.

When the period of active practice is up, carry your practice forward into whatever you do next in your day. Remind yourself to practice for short periods many times throughout the day, and pause from time to time to reflect on how being in the present moment supports your mental health and emotional balance.

AWARENESS PRACTICE #3

Journaling Reflection — Opportunities for Growth

Set aside a period of time, ideally 10 to 20 minutes, for journaling and self-reflection. Remember to bring a sense of warmth, curiosity, and mindful awareness to this and all periods of self-reflection. The point is to get to know your own mind, not to judge what you notice or strive for perfection.

Reflect on your experience over the past 24 hours and explore periods when you were more or less aware and how these periods affected your sense of well-being in the moment. Here are some questions to guide your reflection:

What was I doing and who was I with when I was the most mindful, attentive, or self-aware this past day? How did it feel in this moment? How did it affect what I was doing and my interactions with others?

When was I less mindful, attentive, or self-aware? How did those experiences feel, and how did each affect the quality of my interactions, work, or whatever I was doing at the time?

What is there to learn here? How might I build on the periods where I tend to be more aware and practice the skill of awareness when the awareness meter is down?

Where will I be over the next few days? What will I do and with whom? What would it be like to be fully present and aware in some of these situations? What could I do to make this vision a reality?

AWARENESS PRACTICE #4

Interpersonal Practice—Listening with Mindful Awareness

For this practice, use a conversation or an interaction as a period of practicing the skill of awareness. Begin by setting a clear intention before the interaction begins. It can help to specify a period of time when you are going to make awareness a priority in the interaction. If you'll be with someone for a few hours, for example, it might be challenging to practice for the entire time, but you can make the first 15 minutes a period of formal practice. Then keep up the momentum as best you can for the remaining time.

When you are practicing mindful listening, treat your attention like a gift you are giving the other person. Do your best to be fully present and to notice when your mind is pulled into thoughts. You can still interact and respond as you normally would, but direct some awareness to your own impulses and reactions. Notice if you have a habit of jumping in with a comment before the person is done speaking, or if your habit is simply to hold space when they share something with you. See if you can catch the pull of distraction before it takes hold of your attention, and if you do get distracted, simply celebrate the fact that you noticed and bring your attention back to who you are with.

Beyond any periods of formal practice, when you have a clear intention to use an interaction to practice the skill of awareness, experiment with bringing brief moments of awareness into all your interactions. Notice how being more present and aware affects your relationships with other people.

Additional Practices for the Skill of Connection

CONNECTION PRACTICE #1

Sitting Meditation — Extending Kindness in New Directions

Begin by bringing awareness into your body and find a comfortable, balanced posture. You can keep your eyes gently closed or open in a relaxed gaze, whichever feels more comfortable. As you adjust yourself, notice how small acts like this are an expression of kindness. Here, finding a supportive posture is an act of kindness to yourself.

Next, form a compassionate motivation. Imagine that you are doing this not only for yourself but also to send more kindness and care into the world. Form the aspiration that your practice will genuinely bring more happiness into your life and the lives of others.

Now, rest in open awareness for a few moments. You don't need to do anything, even meditate. Just sit and give yourself a moment to simply exist, to simply be.

Bring to mind someone with whom you have a warm, caring relationship. It could be a friend, a child, or a parent, or even a pet. Imagine that they are sitting here with you and notice the feeling of care and connection you share with them.

Notice your natural and spontaneous wish for this person to be happy and content. This movement toward happiness is kindness. See if you can recognize that in your relationship, both in how you feel toward them and how they feel toward you.

Bring to mind memories and thoughts that bring this shared feeling of mutual kindness into focus. Let your mind roam and steer it toward feelings and thoughts of warmth, affection, and the shared wish that each of you has for the well-being of the other.

If you find it helpful, you can repeat a simple phrase over and over in your mind, something like "May your life be filled with joy" or anything that sparks feelings of kindness.

Now, rest for a moment and notice what you feel in your body. If there are any feelings of warmth or care, savor those feelings, as though you are immersing yourself in the warm glow of kindness. If you don't feel anything special, that's perfectly fine, too. Simply rest your mind in awareness, embracing any feelings or sensations with awareness.

Next, bring to mind someone for whom you don't have strong

feelings, positive or negative. It could be someone you work with but don't know very well, a neighbor, or someone you routinely see at a store.

Imagine that they are here in your presence and that they are a dear friend or loved one. See if you can extend to this person some of the same feelings of kindness and warmth you experienced a few moments ago.

Notice how they want to be happy and free from suffering, just like you and the people you care about.

Imagine scenarios where you might see and interact with them and how you might see them a little differently, perhaps even speak or act with more kindness. What would this look like?

As before, if you find it helpful, you can repeat the phrase "May your life be filled with joy," or another phrase that grounds you in kindness. You can also bring different people to mind and imagine extending them your kind wishes and thoughts.

Conclude by resting in awareness and notice any feelings that are present. If you have feelings of warmth or care, allow those feelings to spread and permeate your entire body. It can help to link this to your breath. As you breathe in and out, imagine that feelings of warmth and connection grow and spread. If no feelings are present, appreciate whatever is happening in your mind and body and rest in a state of effortless presence.

As you transition out of the meditation, use whatever comes next in your day as an opportunity to practice. View every situation as a chance to feel and express kindness, both to yourself and others.

CONNECTION PRACTICE #2

Active Meditation — Commuting with Connection

When we are commuting, traveling, or simply going about our day, we are often surrounded by other people while remaining stuck in our own world. In this practice, you can sharpen the skill of connection by practicing appreciation. The practice here is quite simple. Set aside a specific period of time, which could be your entire trip, or 5, 10, or 15 minutes. For the duration of your practice, find small things to notice and appreciate. It doesn't matter what you notice, or how small. It can be something about yourself or the world around you, but pay special attention to any other people that are present. If you are commuting to work in the morning, for instance, notice the people all around you, whether in other cars or in the same bus or train. Bring to mind positive thoughts: the fact that you are sharing this experience of going somewhere, a nice gesture, a smile, small acts of cooperation. Get creative and see what positive things you can notice. Immerse yourself in the feeling of doing something together. Feel the sense of togetherness as you go wherever it is you are going. Once you arrive, carry on with the practice of appreciation and see if you can notice positive things about every person you meet and interact with.

CONNECTION PRACTICE #3

Writing Reflection— Remembering Compassion

For this journaling reflection, set aside 10 to 20 minutes and reflect on the following questions and prompts:

Think back on your life and recall challenging experiences when you were supported by other people. To begin, don't choose memories that might feel overwhelming. Focus instead on something that feels workable.

What was the experience like? How were you feeling at the time, and who was there to support you? What did this person or these people do or say? How did it feel to know that they were there for you? How did it help you get through this challenging situation?

Now think of a situation where you cared for someone else during a challenging period. What was this situation like? How did you express your feeling of care and compassion? What did you do or say? How did it feel for you to be there for someone in a time of need?

Next, reflect on your life these days. Who might be struggling, whether at work, at home, or anywhere else? How might you extend a helping hand to this person or people? Imagine what it would be like to do so. What would this look like? What might you say or do?

Appendix

CONNECTION PRACTICE # 4

Interpersonal Practice—Warm Memories

For this practice, use a meal with a friend, a loved one, or an entire group to share your warmest memories of connection. Ask each person to share a situation from their life in which they felt the strongest sense of connection with other people and explore together why these situations are so meaningful and supportive of our individual and collective well-being. Share details about the memory itself, how it felt, and also any ripple effect you noticed and may still be aware of.

Additional Practices for the Skill of Insight

INSIGHT PRACTICE #1

Sitting Meditation—Opening to Change

Begin by checking in with your posture and find an upright, relaxed position. You can keep your eyes closed or open with a relaxed gaze, whatever works best for you.

Take a few moments to connect with an inspiring motivation that brings out your very best. Think of the greater good, how doing this practice can bring more insight and wisdom into the world, benefiting you and the people you know and interact with.

Next, let go of any mental effort, even the effort to meditate, and let your mind rest in its natural state. Give yourself some space to simply be.

As you rest in a state of effortless presence, bring a light awareness into your body. You don't need to focus on any one part of your body. Rather, feel the presence of your entire body, as though you are allowing awareness to flow into every pore and cell.

Notice the feelings of movement or change in your body. You may feel a subtle sensation of vibration or the movement of breathing. Notice these changes and allow your awareness to relax into the flow of movement and change, like you are floating downstream in a gentle current.

Now, expand the scope of your attention a bit and take in the world around you. Notice what you hear and see. If your eyes are closed, simply notice the play of light on your eyelids. If they are open, notice the colors and shapes all around you. Listen to the rich array of sounds, including subtle sounds you might normally miss.

Again, notice how your experience of the outside world is changing all the time and relax into the flow of all this change. Welcome it and embrace it with a light touch of awareness.

Next, let go and rest your mind in open awareness. Remain completely open to whatever is happening in your body, mind, and in the world around you. Relax into the shifting, moving flow of experience with a sense of warmth and openness.

For the final step of the practice, bring in some self-reflection by asking yourself, *Where is change happening in my life these days?* Notice what comes to mind, but don't focus on anything too overwhelming. Reflect on things that feel workable.

What thoughts and feelings naturally occur when you bring this situation to mind? Notice how you naturally respond, but without judging what you notice as good or bad.

Now, imagine that you are in touch with your full potential for wisdom and insight. You can see the situation clearly and act wisely. Ask yourself, *How can I view these changes as an opportunity for learning and self-exploration? What is there to learn here?*

As you ask these and other questions, see if you can feel an opening to change and the potential for learning and growth. Feel the confidence of your own potential for insight and see what you notice.

Pause from time to time to notice any feelings or reactions that are present, again without judging them. View everything that happens in your body and mind with a childlike mindset of curiosity.

You can end the meditation by resting in open awareness. Allow any feelings or thoughts to simply flow through your mind. You don't need to indulge them, block them, or change them. Rest in awareness, like the open sky, allowing all the changing weather patterns of your inner experience to come and go like clouds.

When you get up and move on with your day, continue to stay open and curious. Practice short moments of insight by noticing all the change happening within you and around you and staying open to the unpredictable flow of life.

INSIGHT PRACTICE #2

Active Meditation—Thoughts Shape Reality

For this active meditation, pick a period where you are transitioning from one activity to another, ideally a period where you have at least a few minutes in between for some self-inquiry. As you shift gears and move into this activity, notice the inner landscape of your thoughts and emotions. What thoughts are moving through your mind? What feelings and emotions are present in your body? No need to judge what you notice as right or wrong, or good or bad. The point here is to get curious and explore your inner landscape.

Once you've noticed your mental and emotional state, ask yourself, *How are my thoughts and feelings shaping the way I see things right now, and how will I experience the situation I'm moving into?* Again, no need for judgment here. The point is to explore and gain insight into the workings of your own mind. If you notice a stream of stressed-out thoughts, for example, you might see that they are prompting you to fixate on something negative and to ignore positive things. If your mind is distracted, you may see that you are simply not taking in everything that is happening because you are up in your head and lost in thought. Whatever you find, bring a sense of playful curiosity to your inner experience, as if you were a small child trying to understand your own mind and how it works.

INSIGHT PRACTICE #3

Writing Reflection — What Leads to Growth and Insight?

For the following journaling exercise, set aside a period of time to sit and reflect on an important period of growth and learning, and use this reflection to see your current life circumstances in a new light.

When you look back on your life, what stands out as a period where you learned a lot about yourself and grew as an individual?

What circumstances supported your ability to learn and grow? What was going on within you that made this possible? What thoughts, perspectives, or inner factors supported you in this period?

What is going on in your life these days that might provide a similar opportunity for inner exploration and growth? How might you bring some of the same perspectives or other factors to bear on this situation? How might you set yourself up for new insights to take root in your mind?

INSIGHT PRACTICE #4

Interpersonal Practice—Exploring the Web of Causes and Conditions

This practice can be done with a friend or a partner. Each person takes a turn sharing and a turn listening. When sharing, pick a situation in your life that feels important, in either a positive or a negative way, but nothing too overwhelming. Start by sharing a bit about the situation and how you feel about it. Next, dig deeper and share all the influences and circumstances that shape both the situation and how you experience it. The listener can probe deeper from time to time, prompting more reflection on all the many causes and conditions that are manifest in this situation. After a period of time, usually 5 to 10 minutes, switch roles.

Additional Practices for the Skill of Purpose

PURPOSE PRACTICE #1

Sitting Meditation—Meaningful Memories

For the first few minutes of your practice, bring awareness into your body and find a posture that supports a wakeful, relaxed presence. You can keep your eyes open, with a relaxed gaze, or gently close them. Once you feel settled, take a few moments to form an inspiring motivation to guide your meditation. See if you can link your practice to a sense of purpose that feels meaningful and uplifting.

Next, pause for a minute or two and rest in open awareness. When resting in open awareness, you don't need to focus or concentrate. Simply be. Rest in your natural state, however that may feel in the present moment.

Now, to practice the skill of purpose, bring to mind an experience from your life that feels especially meaningful or fulfilling. Bring yourself back to that experience and see if you can remember some of the details and how it felt.

Ask yourself, *Why was this experience so meaningful?* As you reflect on this question, see if you can find a connection between the experience and a guiding purpose or principle in your life that feels important. The purpose could be anything, even something as simple as wanting to be there for the people you care about. Reflect with curiosity and an attitude of playful experimentation. There are no right or wrong answers. Just explore and see what you notice.

Once you've uncovered a deeper purpose or an important personal value or principle, explore other experiences and memories. Where has this purpose shown up in other areas of your life? When do you feel most connected to this perspective and worldview?

For the final step, think about your current life. Where do you see this sense of purpose manifesting in your life right now? Where do you see opportunities to stay aligned with this purpose?

Throughout the period of self-reflection, you can alternate between periods of contemplation and periods of resting in open awareness.

Conclude your practice with a minute or two of resting in open awareness. Allow your mind to rest in its natural state and bring a sense of warmth and appreciation to whatever arises in the field of your awareness.

As you transition out of the practice, keep your sense of purpose clearly in mind. See if you can link whatever you do next to something you find meaningful and fulfilling, and bring short moments of purpose into the flow of your daily routine.

PURPOSE PRACTICE #2

Active Meditation—Finding Meaning in the Mundane

To practice the skill of purpose as an active meditation you can do in everyday life, pick a boring activity that's part of your daily routine, like washing the dishes or doing the laundry. Do the activity as you would any other day but add some depth and meaning to the process. You can do this by asking yourself why you are actually doing the task or activity. Every time you come up with an answer, probe a little deeper and ask why again, until you find something linked to a deeper sense of purpose. For instance, if you ask yourself, *Why am I doing the dishes right now?* you might answer, *Well, because I don't want my kitchen to be a mess.* Then, dig deeper and ask, *Why don't I want my kitchen to be dirty?* If you live alone, the inquiry might help you to see that you feel more calm and relaxed in a tidy home, and that your deeper desire is to feel truly at home.

If you live with others, you might want your home to be clean so your loved ones or roommates enjoy being there, and if you probe even deeper, you may see that you want that because you care about them.

With this new perspective, you can see that one of your deeper motivations for doing the dishes is love and your care for others. You could then take one more step and see that by doing the dishes and linking what you are doing to a deeper purpose (such as wanting the people in your life to feel loved), you are part of a much larger movement of countless people expressing love. Now, your seemingly boring chore is part of a global current of love in the world.

You can do this practice with any activity. The key is to stay open and curious. You may hit a dead end when you probe and explore. If you do, just back up and try a new line of inquiry. Eventually, you will be able to find meaning and purpose in any activity, no matter how mundane or meaningless it may seem.

Appendix

PURPOSE PRACTICE #3

Writing Reflection—Planning on Purpose

For this journaling reflection, set aside 5 to 15 minutes, or longer if you prefer, and sketch out a simple plan to practice the skill of purpose over the next few days. You can use the following prompts to guide your reflection.

Pick a guiding purpose or principle to explore in your experience over the next few days. It should be something that will be broad enough that you can apply it in many situations, like kindness or integrity. Begin your reflection by exploring what this particular principle means to you and why you chose to focus on it.

Next, make a plan. Pick one activity per day over the next few days that you can link to your guiding purpose. Note when and where the activity will happen and how you will remember to practice.

For each activity, be specific. How will you remind yourself to use the activity as an opportunity to practice? Will you practice the skill of purpose simply by changing your perspective on the activity? Will you do or say anything different? Be creative and explore new ways to link everyday activities with a deeper sense of purpose.

Appendix

PURPOSE PRACTICE #4

Interpersonal Practice—
100th Birthday Party

To explore the skill of purpose in conversation, brainstorm with a close friend or a loved one what your 100th birthday party might be like. Imagine you are looking back on your entire life, surrounded by people you love. Each person is sharing something about you and your life that they respect, admire, or appreciate. What would you want them to say? What impact will you have had on their lives and the lives of others? Let your imagination roam and see what rises to the surface that feels most meaningful. Each person can take a turn sharing a vision for their own 100th birthday party. Once you have both shared, you can talk about how it went and what you learned, especially what pertains to your guiding principles and purpose.

RESOURCES

The Healthy Minds Program

The Healthy Minds Program is a guided path to training the mind based on the Healthy Minds Framework and the four dimensions of awareness, connection, insight, and purpose. This program is available as a free mobile app with hundreds of guided meditations, podcast-style lessons, and tips for applying the four skills in a range of daily life situations. Hundreds of thousands of people have used the Healthy Minds Program to cultivate well-being. If you found the insights and practices we wrote about here helpful, we highly recommend downloading the app to learn more and deepen your experience.

The Center for Healthy Minds (CHM)

The Center for Healthy Minds is an interdisciplinary research center founded by Richie at the University of Wisconsin–Madison in 2009. The mission of the Center is to cultivate well-being and relieve suffering through a scientific understanding of the mind. The Center employs approximately seventy people and includes twelve core faculty. The Center conducts both basic and translational research and engages in educational and community outreach activities. More information can be found at www.centerhealthyminds.org.

Appendix

Humin

Humin (formerly Healthy Minds Innovations) is a nonprofit corporation that was founded by Richie in 2014. He was moved to create this nonprofit in recognition of the need to bring our insights from the science into the world. Richie experienced this as a moral calling, a mandate to be an activist scientist. The mission of Humin is to take the insights from the science and turn them into tools that can be used to measure and cultivate well-being. Humin is the organization behind our mobile app, the Healthy Minds Program. More information about Humin can be found at www.humin.org.

Tergar International

Tergar International, which Cort cofounded in 2009 with Yongey Mingyur Rinpoche, oversees a global meditation community designed to make profound meditation practices accessible to everyone. Tergar offers a complete pathway of meditation training—from simple mindfulness techniques to deep explorations of the nature of consciousness. Their approach balances ancient wisdom with modern science, creating programs that resonate with people of all backgrounds and beliefs. Through online courses, in-person retreats, and local practice groups across six continents, Tergar provides both structure for beginners and depth for experienced practitioners. Thousands have discovered how these practices can transform their relationship with life's challenges. Explore their offerings at www.tergar.org.

Notes

Chapter 1: What Flourishing Is and Why It Matters

10 *We will share our groundbreaking scientific model—the Healthy Minds Framework*: C. J. Dahl, C. D. Wilson-Mendenhall, and R. J. Davidson, "The Plasticity of Well-Being: A Training-Based Framework for the Cultivation of Human Flourishing," *Proceedings of the National Academy of Sciences* 117, no. 51 (2020): 32197–206, https://doi.org/10.1073/pnas.2014859117.

12 *Scientists call this the "declarative-procedural gap"*: A. Demir, M. Kiziloglu, T. Budur, and A. Heshmati, "Elaborating on the Links Between Declarative Knowledge, Procedural Knowledge, and Employee Performance," *SN Business & Economics* 3, no. 1 (2022), http://doi.org/10.1007/s43546-022-00402-3.

13 *doing the practices we teach in this book for just five minutes a day*: M. J. Hirshberg, C. Frye, C. J. Dahl, K. M. Riordan, N. J. Vack, J. Sachs, R. Goldman, R. J. Davidson, and S. B. Goldberg, "A Randomized Controlled Trial of a Smartphone-Based Well-Being Training in Public School System Employees During the COVID-19 Pandemic," *Journal of Educational Psychology* 114, no. 8 (2022):1895–1911, http://doi.org/10.1037/edu0000739. Epub March 17, 2022.

14 *we taught people who had never done any form of meditation training a simple compassion practice*: H. Y. Weng, A. S. Fox, A. J. Shackman, D. E. Stodola, J. Z. K. Caldwell, M. C. Olson, G. M. Rogers, and R. J. Davidson, "Compassion Training Alters Altruism and Neural Responses to Suffering," *Psychological Science* 24, no. 7 (2013): 1171–80, https://doi.org/10.1177/0956797612469537.

15 *showing significant gains in measures of well-being*: A. Malaktaris, A. J. Lang, P. Casmar, S. Baca, S. Hurst, D. v. Jeste, and B. W. Palmer, "Pilot Study of Compassion Meditation Training to Improve Well-Being Among Older Adults," *Clinical Gerontologist* 45, no. 2 (2022), 287–300, https://doi.org/10.1080/07317115.2020.1839826.

15 *Advanced meditators had much less activity in the pain network*: A. Lutz, D. R. McFarlin, D. M. Perlman, T. v. Salomons, and R. J. Davidson, "Altered Anterior Insula Activation During Anticipation and Experience of Painful Stimuli

in Expert Meditators," *NeuroImage* 64 (2013): 538–46, https://doi.org/10.1016/j.neuroimage.2012.09.030.

Chapter 2: Rewiring Your Brain to Flourish

25 *Neuroplasticity*: For a good overview of both neuroplasticity and epigenetics and how they are relevant to flourishing, see Bruce S. McEwen, "In Pursuit of Resilience: Stress, Epigenetics, and Brain Plasticity," *Annals of the New York Academy of Sciences* 1373, no. 1 (2016): 56–64, https://doi.org/10.1111/nyas.13020.

25 *The next time you try to juggle will be easier*: For review, see Jan Scholz, Miriam C. Klein, Timothy E. J. Behrens, and Heidi Johansen-Berg, "Training Induces Changes in White-Matter Architecture," *Nature Neuroscience* 12, no. 11 (2009): 1370–71, https://doi.org/10.1038/nn.2412.

25 *Epigenetics*: Ibid.

25 *This decrease in inflammation, a common factor in many chronic illnesses*: R. Chaix, M. Fagny, M. Cosin-Tomás, M. Alvarez-López, L. Lemee, B. Regnault, R. J. Davidson, A. Lutz, and P. Kaliman, "Differential DNA Methylation in Experienced Meditators After an Intensive Day of Mindfulness-Based Practice: Implications for Immune-Related Pathways," *Brain, Behavior, and Immunity* 84 (February 2020): 36–44, https://doi.org/10.1016/j.bbi.2019.11.003.

28 *The insula is the only part of the brain that contains what we call a "viscerotopic map"*: C. Stephani, G. Fernandez-Baca Vaca, R. MacIunas, M. Koubeissi, and H. O. Lüders, "Functional Neuroanatomy of the Insular Lobe," *Brain Structure and Function* 216, no. 2 (2011): 137–49, https://doi.org/10.1007/s00429-010-0296-3.

28 *when your brain perceives the acceleration of your breathing and heart rate*: William James, "The Physical Basis of Emotion," *Psychological Review* 101 (1994).

30 *Researchers were particularly interested in the hippocampus*: E. A. Maguire, D. G. Gadian, I. S. Johnsrude, C. D. Good, J. Ashburner, R. S. J. Frackowiak, and C. D. Frith, "Navigation-Related Structural Change in the Hippocampi of Taxi Drivers," *Proceedings of the National Academy of Sciences* 97, no. 8 (2000): 4398, http://www.pnas.org/content/97/8/4398.short.

31 *possible changes in the neuronal connections between different brain regions*: Tammi R. A. Kral, Kaley Davis, Cole Korponay, Matthew J. Hirshberg, Rachel Hoel, Lawrence Y. Tello, Robin I. Goldman, Melissa A. Rosenkranz, Antoine Lutz, and Richard J. Davidson, "Absence of Structural Brain Changes from Mindfulness-Based Stress Reduction: Two Combined Randomized Controlled Trials," *Science Advances* 8, no. 20 (2022), https://doi.org/10.1126/sciadv.abk3316.

31 *Health Enhancement Program, a training we invented to control for the group experience*: Donal G. MacCoon, Zac E. Imel, Melissa A. Rosenkranz, Jenna G. Sheftel, Helen Y. Weng, Jude C. Sullivan, Katherine A. Bonus et al., "The Validation of an Active Control Intervention for Mindfulness Based Stress Reduction (MBSR),"

Behaviour Research and Therapy 50, no. 1 (2012): 3–12, https://doi.org/10.1016/j.brat.2011.10.011.

33 *have a less severe presentation of the illness*: Lucia Migliore and Fabio Coppedè, "Gene–Environment Interactions in Alzheimer Disease: The Emerging Role of Epigenetics," *Nature Reviews Neurology* 18 (2022): 643–60, https://doi.org/10.1038/s41582-022-00714-w.

34 *groundbreaking article about the epigenetics of stress*: Rachel Yehuda, Nikolaos P. Daskalakis, Linda M. Bierer, Heather N. Bader, Torsten Klengel, Florian Holsboer, and Elisabeth B. Binder, "Holocaust Exposure Induced Intergenerational Effects on FKBP5 Methylation," *Biological Psychiatry* 80, no. 5 (2016): 372–80, https://doi.org/10.1016/j.biopsych.2015.08.005.

35 *a novel study with 19 long-term meditation practitioners*: Perla Kaliman, María Jesús Álvarez-López, Marta Cosín-Tomás, Melissa A. Rosenkranz, Antoine Lutz, and Richard J. Davidson, "Rapid Changes in Histone Deacetylases and Inflammatory Gene Expression in Expert Meditators," *Psychoneuroendocrinology* 40 (2014): 96–107, http://www.sciencedirect.com/science/article/pii/S0306453013004071.

38 *One body of work has shown that infants are oriented toward kindness*: J. K. Hamlin, "Moral Judgment and Action in Preverbal Infants and Toddlers: Evidence for an Innate Moral Core," *Current Directions in Psychological Science* 22, no. 3 (2013): 186–93, https://doi.org/10.1177/0963721412470687.

38 *experiment in which six-month-old infants sat on their mother's lap*: J. Kiley Hamlin, Karen Wynn, and Paul Bloom, "Social Evaluation by Preverbal Infants," *Nature* 450, no. 7169 (2007): 557–59, https://doi.org/10.1038/nature06288.

39 *three characteristics of infants that convincingly reveal our innate capacity to flourish*: J. K. Hamlin, "Moral Judgment and Action in Preverbal Infants and Toddlers: Evidence for an Innate Moral Core," *Current Directions in Psychological Science* 22, no. 3 (2013): 186–93, https://doi.org/10.1177/0963721412470687.

Chapter 3: Flourishing in the Midst of Challenge

46 *has described this premature mortality as "deaths of despair"*: Anne Case and Angus Deaton, "Rising Morbidity and Mortality in Midlife Among White Non-Hispanic Americans in the 21st Century," *Proceedings of the National Academy of Sciences* 112, no. 49 (2015): 15078–83, https://doi.org/10.1073/pnas.1518393112.

46 *when we're not aware of the factors influencing us, it's very difficult to regulate our responses*: Regina C. Lapate, Bas Rokers, Tianyi Li, and Richard J. Davidson, "Nonconscious Emotional Activation Colors First Impressions," *Psychological Science* 25, no. 2 (2014): 349–57, https://doi.org/10.1177/0956797613503175.

47 *some findings even showing abnormalities in brain regions*: Juliane Horvath, Christina Mundinger, Mike M. Schmitgen, Nadine D. Wolf, Fabio Sambataro, Dusan Hirjak, Katharina M. Kubera, Julian Koenig, and Robert

Christian Wolf, "Structural and Functional Correlates of Smartphone Addiction," *Addictive Behaviors* 105 (January 2020): 106334, https://doi.org/10.1016/j.addbeh.2020.106334.

48 *500 adult participants were asked to reduce their smartphone use*: Lena Marie Precht, Franziska Mertens, Debora S. Brickau, Romy J. Kramm, Jürgen Margraf, Jan Stirnberg, and Julia Brailovskaia, "Engaging in Physical Activity Instead of (over) Using the Smartphone: An Experimental Investigation of Lifestyle Interventions to Prevent Problematic Smartphone Use and to Promote Mental Health," *Journal of Public Health (Germany)* 32, no. 4 (2024): 589–607, https://doi.org/10.1007/s10389-023-01832-5.

49 *an innovative method called "experience sampling"*: M. A. Killingsworth and D. T. Gilbert, "A Wandering Mind Is an Unhappy Mind," *Science* 330, no. 6006 (2010): 932, https://doi.org/10.1126/science.1192439.

52 *Presenting sobering evidence for significant downward trends in social connection*: U.S. Surgeon General, "Our Epidemic of Loneliness and Isolation," (2023): 1–82, https://www.hhs.gov/sites/default/files/surgeon-general-social-connection-advisory.pdf.

53 *Social isolation also compromises our insula*: Yajie Zhang, Sai Ma, Youyi Liu, Feng Kong, and Zonglei Zhen, "Functional Integration of Anterior Insula Related to Meaning in Life and Loneliness," *Journal of Affective Disorders* 338 (October 2023): 10–16, https://doi.org/10.1016/j.jad.2023.05.067; Niccolò Zovetti, Maria Gloria Rossetti, Cinzia Perlini, Paolo Brambilla, and Marcella Bellani, "Neuroimaging Studies Exploring the Neural Basis of Social Isolation," *Epidemiology and Psychiatric Sciences* 30 (2021), https://doi.org/10.1017/S2045796021000135.

56 *studied the relationship between money and flourishing in novel ways*: Andrew T. Jebb, Louis Tay, Ed Diener, and Shigehiro Oishi, "Happiness, Income Satiation and Turning Points Around the World," *Nature Human Behaviour* 2, no. 1 (2018): 33–38, https://doi.org/10.1038/s41562-017-0277-0. The relationship between money and happiness has generated much conflicting evidence, largely due to how "happiness" or flourishing is assessed. When hedonic happiness is measured, the satiation point found by Oishi is present only for the least happy people. See Matthew A. Killingsworth, Daniel Kahneman, and Barbara Mellers, "Income and Emotional Well-Being: A Conflict Resolved," *Proceedings of the National Academy of Sciences* 120, no. 10 (2023), https://doi.org/10.1073/pnas.2208661120.

58 *Jamie Hanson has led much of the work on trauma at the Center for Healthy Minds*: Jamie L. Hanson, Nagesh Adluru, Moo K. Chung, Andrew L. Alexander, Richard J. Davidson, and Seth D. Pollak, "Early Neglect Is Associated with Alterations in White Matter Integrity and Cognitive Functioning," *Child Development* 84, no. 5 (2013): 1566–78, https://doi.org/10.1111/cdev.12069; L. Hanson, Wouter van den Bos, Barbara J. Roeber, Karen D. Rudolph, Richard J. Davidson, and Seth D. Pollak, "Early Adversity and Learning: Implications for Typical and Atypical

Behavioral Development," *Journal of Child Psychology and Psychiatry* 58, no. 7 (2017): 770–78, https://doi.org/10.1111/jcpp.12694; Jamie L. Hanson, Moo K. Chung, Brian B. Avants, Karen D. Rudolph, Elizabeth A. Shirtcliff, James C. Gee, Richard J. Davidson, and Seth D. Pollak, "Structural Variations in Prefrontal Cortex Mediate the Relationship Between Early Childhood Stress and Spatial Working Memory," *Journal of Neuroscience* 32, no. 23 (2012): 7917–25, https://doi.org/10.1523/JNEUROSCI.0307-12.2012; Jamie L. Hanson, Moo K. Chung, Brian B. Avants, Elizabeth A. Shirtcliff, James C. Gee, Richard J. Davidson, and Seth D. Pollak, "Early Stress Is Associated with Alterations in the Orbitofrontal Cortex: A Tensor-Based Morphometry Investigation of Brain Structure and Behavioral Risk," *Journal of Neuroscience* 30, no. 22 (2010): 7466–72, https://doi.org/10.1523/JNEUROSCI.0859-10.2010; L. Hanson, Brendon M. Nacewicz, Matthew J. Sutterer, Amelia A. Cayo, Stacey M. Schaefer, Karen D. Rudolph, Elizabeth A. Shirtcliff, Seth D. Pollak, and Richard J. Davidson, "Behavioral Problems After Early Life Stress: Contributions of the Hippocampus and Amygdala," *Biological Psychiatry* 77, no. 4 (2015): 314–23, https://doi.org/10.1016/j.biopsych.2014.04.020.

59 *Andrea Danese of the Institute of Psychiatry at King's College in London and his colleague Cathy Widom*: Andrea Danese and Cathy Spatz Widom, "Objective and Subjective Experiences of Child Maltreatment and Their Relationships with Psychopathology," *Nature Human Behaviour* 4, no. 8 (2020): 811–18, https://doi.org/10.1038/s41562-020-0880-3.

60 *an intensive intervention to promote flourishing skills had a dramatic impact on their ability to heal*: Perla Kaliman, Marta Cosín-Tomás, Andy Madrid, Susana Roque López, Elkin Llanez-Anaya, Ligia A. Papale, Reid S. Alisch, and Richard J. Davidson, "Epigenetic Impact of a 1-Week Intensive Multimodal Group Program for Adolescents with Multiple Adverse Childhood Experiences," *Scientific Reports* 12, no. 1 (2022): 17177, https://doi.org/10.1038/s41598-022-21246-9.

62 *He cross-fostered the young rats from the high- and low-anxious groups*: Tie-Yuan Zhang and Michael J. Meaney, "Epigenetics and the Environmental Regulation of the Genome and Its Function," *Annual Review of Psychology* 61 (January 2010): 439–66, C1–3, https://doi.org/10.1146/annurev.psych.60.110707.163625.

Chapter 4: The Path to Flourishing

69 *The two most influential models focus on "hedonic" and "eudaimonic" well-being*: Richard M. Ryan and Edward L. Deci, "On Happiness and Human Potentials: A Review of Research on Hedonic and Eudaimonic Well-Being," *Annual Review of Psychology* 52 (2001): 141–66.

69 *scientists formed different models of human flourishing*: Antonella Delle Fave, "Eudaimonic and Hedonic Happiness," in *Encyclopedia of Quality of Life and*

Well-Being Research, Springer International Publishing (2021): 1–7, https://doi.org/10.1007/978-3-319-69909-7_3778-2.

75 *impacted basic biological functions like their spontaneous eyeblink rate*: Ayla Kruis, Heleen A. Slagter, David R. W. Bachhuber, Richard J. Davidson, and Antoine Lutz, "Effects of Meditation Practice on Spontaneous Eyeblink Rate," *Psychophysiology* 53, no. 5 (2016): 749–58, https://doi.org/10.1111/psyp.12619.

77 *He almost died from food poisoning*: Yongey Mingyur Rinpoche, *In Love with the World: A Monk's Journey Through the Bardos of Living and Dying* (New York: Random House, 2019).

78 *you would have no way of knowing that these meditators were in a state of deep concentration*: J. A. Brefczynski-Lewis, A. Lutz, H. S. Schaefer, D. B. Levinson, and R. J. Davidson, "Neural Correlates of Attentional Expertise in Long-Term Meditation Practitioners," *Proceedings of the National Academy of Sciences* 104, no. 27 (2007): 11483–88, https://doi.org/10.1073/pnas.0606552104.

82 *Scientific research on well-being has long focused on positive social interactions and strong relationships*: Annie Regan, Nina Radošić, and Sonja Lyubomirsky, "Experimental Effects of Social Behavior on Well-Being," *Trends in Cognitive Sciences* 26, no. 11 (2022): 987–98, https://doi.org/10.1016/j.tics.2022.08.006.

84 *The Way of a Pilgrim, a book from the Russian Orthodox Christian tradition*: Anonymous, translated by Olga Savin, *The Way of a Pilgrim* (Boulder, CO: Shambhala, 2001).

87 *publication in the prestigious* Proceedings of the National Academy of Sciences *in 2020*: Cortland J. Dahl, Christine D. Wilson-Mendenhall, and Richard J. Davidson, "The Plasticity of Well-Being: A Training-Based Framework for the Cultivation of Human Flourishing," *Proceedings of the National Academy of Sciences* 117, no. 51 (2020): 32197–206, https://doi.org/10.1073/pnas.2014859117.

88 *scientific tool to measure the four skills of awareness, connection, insight, and purpose—the Healthy Minds Index*: Tammi R. A. Kral, Pelin Kesebir, Liz Redford, Cortland J. Dahl, Christine D. Wilson-Mendenhall, Matthew J. Hirshberg, Richard J. Davidson, and Raquel Tatar, "Healthy Minds Index: A Brief Measure of the Core Dimensions of Well-Being," *PloS One* 19, no. 5 (2024): e0299352, https://doi.org/10.1371/journal.pone.0299352.

94 *You can train your mind in just minutes a day*: Matthew J. Hirshberg, Corrina Frye, Cortland J. Dahl, Kevin M. Riordan, Nathan J. Vack, Jane Sachs, Robin Goldman, Richard J. Davidson, and Simon B. Goldberg, "A Randomized Controlled Trial of a Smartphone-Based Well-Being Training in Public School System Employees During the COVID-19 Pandemic," *Journal of Educational Psychology* 114, no. 8 (March 2022): 1895–1911, https://doi.org/10.1037/edu0000739.

Notes

Chapter 5: Awareness: The First Skill of Flourishing

98 *it confirmed their hypothesis that advanced meditators respond to pain differently*: Antoine Lutz, Daniel R. McFarlin, David M. Perlman, Tim v. Salomons, and Richard J. Davidson, "Altered Anterior Insula Activation During Anticipation and Experience of Painful Stimuli in Expert Meditators," *NeuroImage* 64 (January 2013): 538–46, https://doi.org/10.1016/j.neuroimage.2012.09.030.

102 *we define awareness as "a heightened and flexible attentiveness" to what is happening in the moment*: Cortland J. Dahl, Christine D. Wilson-Mendenhall, and Richard J. Davidson, "The Plasticity of Well-Being: A Training-Based Framework for the Cultivation of Human Flourishing," *Proceedings of the National Academy of Sciences* 117, no. 51 (2020): 32197–206, https://doi.org/10.1073/pnas.2014859117.

104 *were able to activate the same brain networks linked to attention and awareness that the experts activated*: Tammi R. A. Kral, Ted Imhoff-Smith, Douglas C. Dean, Dan Grupe, Nagesh Adluru, Elena Patsenko, Jeanette A. Mumford, Robin Goldman, Melissa A. Rosenkranz, and Richard J. Davidson, "Mindfulness-Based Stress Reduction-Related Changes in Posterior Cingulate Resting Brain Connectivity," *Social Cognitive and Affective Neuroscience* 14, no. 7 (2019): 777–87, https://doi.org/10.1093/scan/nsz050.

108 *we referred to the movement from distraction to awareness as a shift from "experiential fusion" to "meta-awareness"*: Cortland J. Dahl, Antoine Lutz, and Richard J. Davidson, "Reconstructing and Deconstructing the Self: Cognitive Mechanisms in Meditation Practice," *Trends in Cognitive Sciences* 19, no. 9 (2015): 515–23, https://doi.org/10.1016/j.tics.2015.07.001.

110 *the experience of being so completely focused on a particular activity and absorbed in the moment*: J. Nakamura and M. Csikszentmihalyi, "The Concept of Flow," in *Flow and the Foundations of Positive Psychology*, edited by M. Csikszentmihalyi (Dordrecht: Springer, 2014), https://www.researchgate.net/publication/372282514.

111 *we find all the ingredients we need to build a strong awareness practice*: Jon Kabat-Zinn, *Wherever You Go, There You Are: Mindfulness Meditation in Everyday Life* (New York: Hyperion, 1994).

117 *we recruited a group of 40 experienced meditators to measure how the brain changes with awareness practice*: Tammi R. A. Kral, Regina C. Lapate, Ted Imhoff-Smith, Elena Patsenko, Daniel W. Grupe, Robin Goldman, Melissa A. Rosenkranz, and Richard J. Davidson, "Long-Term Meditation Training Is Associated with Enhanced Subjective Attention and Stronger Posterior Cingulate–Rostrolateral Prefrontal Cortex Resting Connectivity," *Journal of Cognitive Neuroscience* 34, no. 9 (2022): 1576–89, https://doi.org/10.1162/jocn_a_01881.

118 *In another study, we recruited roughly 150 subjects and put them into three groups*: Tammi R. A. Kral, Brianna S. Schuyler, Jeanette A. Mumford, Melissa A. Rosenkranz, Antoine Lutz, and Richard J. Davidson, "Impact of Short- and

Long-Term Mindfulness Meditation Training on Amygdala Reactivity to Emotional Stimuli," *NeuroImage* 181 (November 2018): 301–13, https://doi.org/10.1016/j.neuroimage.2018.07.013.

Chapter 6: Connection: The Second Skill of Flourishing

126 *More important is how you feel about your relationships, particularly how supported you feel*: Caitlin E. Coyle and Elizabeth Dugan, "Social Isolation, Loneliness and Health Among Older Adults," *Journal of Aging and Health* 24, no. 8 (2012): 1346–63, https://doi.org/10.1177/0898264312460275; John T. Cacioppo and Stephanie Cacioppo, "Social Relationships and Health: The Toxic Effects of Perceived Social Isolation," *Social and Personality Psychology Compass* 8, no. 2 (2014): 58–72, https://doi.org/10.1111/spc3.12087.

127 *no matter how lonely and isolated our circumstances might be, we can still cultivate a sense of connection*: Matthew J. Hirshberg, Corrina Frye, Cortland J. Dahl, Kevin M. Riordan, Nathan J. Vack, Jane Sachs, Robin Goldman, Richard J. Davidson, and Simon B. Goldberg, "A Randomized Controlled Trial of a Smartphone-Based Well-Being Training in Public School System Employees During the COVID-19 Pandemic," *Journal of Educational Psychology* 114, no. 8 (2022): 1895–1911, https://doi.org/10.1037/edu0000739.

129 *Feeling connected even supports our immune system*: Keely A. Muscatell, "Social Psychoneuroimmunology: Understanding Bidirectional Links Between Social Experiences and the Immune System," *Brain, Behavior, and Immunity* 93 (2021): 1–3, https://doi.org/10.1016/j.bbi.2020.12.023.

138 *these practices can reduce unconscious bias in the classroom and that the effects don't disappear after training ends*: Matthew J. Hirshberg, Lisa Flook, Evan E. Moss, Robert D. Enright, and Richard J. Davidson, "Integrating Mindfulness and Connection Practices into Preservice Teacher Education Results in Durable Automatic Race Bias Reductions," *Journal of School Psychology* 91 (April 2022): 50–64, https://doi.org/10.1016/j.jsp.2021.12.002.

138 *teachers were more likely to still be teaching three years later*: Matthew J. Hirshberg, Lisa Flook, Reka Sundaram-Stukel, and Richard J. Davidson, "Mindfulness and Connection Training During Preservice Teacher Education Reduces Early Career Teacher Attrition 4 Years Later," *Journal of School Psychology* 107 (December 2024): 101396, https://doi.org/10.1016/j.jsp.2024.101396.

142 *completely different experiences that activate entirely different brain networks*: Tania Singer and Olga M. Klimecki, "Empathy and Compassion," *Current Biology* 24, no. 18 (2014): R875–78, https://doi.org/10.1016/j.cub.2014.06.054.

143 *Dr. Helen Weng was the lead scientist on this study*: Helen Y. Weng, Andrew S. Fox, Alexander J. Shackman, Diane E. Stodola, Jessica Z. K. Caldwell, Matthew C. Olson, Gregory M. Rogers, and Richard J. Davidson, "Compassion Training

Alters Altruism and Neural Responses to Suffering," *Psychological Science* 24, no. 7 (2013): 1171–80, https://doi.org/10.1177/0956797612469537.

Chapter 7: Insight: The Third Skill of Flourishing

153   *patients who were able to step back and examine their own beliefs and perceptions tended to do better in treatment*: For a good review of cognitive insight, see L. S. C. van Camp, B. G. C. Sabbe, and J. F. E. Oldenburg, "Cognitive Insight: A Systematic Review," *Clinical Psychology Review* 55 (March 2017): 12–24, https://doi.org/10.1016/j.cpr.2017.04.011.

153   *developed a scientifically validated questionnaire to measure it*: Aaron T. Beck, Edward Baruch, Jordan M. Balter, Robert A. Steer, and Debbie M. Warman, "A New Instrument for Measuring Insight: The Beck Cognitive Insight Scale," *Schizophrenia Research* 68, no. 2–3 (2004): 319–29, https://doi.org/10.1016/S0920-9964(03)00189-0.

160   *self-inquiry does indeed strengthen our ability to regulate our emotional reactions in new and healthy ways*: Lea K. Hilderbrandt, C. McCall, and T. Singer, "Socioaffective Versus Sociocognitive Mental Trainings Differentially Affect Emotion Regulation Strategies," *Emotion* 19, no. 8 (2019): 132942, https://doi.org/10.1037/emo0000518.supp.

160   *we replicated a growing body of research that shows how cultivating insight and other dimensions of flourishing through meditation training*: Tammi R. A. Kral, Regina C. Lapate, Ted Imhoff-Smith, Elena Patsenko, Daniel W. Grupe, Robin Goldman, Melissa A. Rosenkranz, and Richard J. Davidson, "Long-Term Meditation Training Is Associated with Enhanced Subjective Attention and Stronger Posterior Cingulate–Rostrolateral Prefrontal Cortex Resting Connectivity," *Journal of Cognitive Neuroscience* 34, no. 9 (2022): 1576–89, https://doi.org/10.1162/jocn_a_01881.

169   *we examined them during different styles of practice, measuring the electrical activity in their brains with an EEG*: A. Lutz, L. L. Greischar, N. B. Rawlings, M. Ricard, and R. J. Davidson, "Long-Term Meditators Self-Induce High-Amplitude Gamma Synchrony During Mental Practice," *Proceedings of the National Academy of Sciences* 101, no. 46 (2004): 16369–73, https://doi.org/10.1073/pnas.0407401101.

Chapter 8: Purpose: The Fourth Skill of Flourishing

183   *In an influential framework created by our colleague Carol Ryff*: Carol D. Ryff and Corey Lee M. Keyes, "The Structure of Psychological Well-Being Revisited," *Journal of Personality and Social Psychology* 69, no. 4 (1995): 719–27, https://doi.org/10.1037/0022-3514.69.4.719.

184   *and a lower risk of stroke*: Eric S. Kim, Jennifer K. Sun, Nansook Park, and Christopher Peterson, "Purpose in Life and Reduced Incidence of Stroke in Older

Adults: 'The Health and Retirement Study,'" *Journal of Psychosomatic Research* 74, no. 5 (2013): 427–32, https://doi.org/10.1016/j.jpsychores.2013.01.013. For a more recent overview of this area, see Eric S. Kim, Ying Chen, Julia S. Nakamura, Carol D. Ryff, and Tyler J. VanderWeele, "Sense of Purpose in Life and Subsequent Physical, Behavioral, and Psychosocial Health: An Outcome-Wide Approach," *American Journal of Health Promotion* 36, no. 1 (2022): 137–47, https://doi.org/10.1177/08901171211038545.

184 *a strong sense of purpose supports healthy aging*: Ajay Kumar Nair, Nagesh Adluru, Anna J. Finley, Lauren K. Gresham, Sarah E. Skinner, Andrew L. Alexander, Richard J. Davidson, Carol D. Ryff, and Stacey M. Schaefer, "Purpose in Life as a Resilience Factor for Brain Health: Diffusion MRI Findings from the Midlife in the U.S. Study," *Frontiers in Psychiatry* 15 (2024): 1–12, https://doi.org/10.3389/fpsyt.2024.1355998.

187 *if kids see their educational journey in light of their most important values and guiding principles*: J. Parker Goyer, Julio Garcia, Valerie Purdie-Vaughns, Kevin R. Binning, Jonathan E. Cook, Stephanie L. Reeves, Nancy Apfel, Suzanne Taborsky-Barba, David K. Sherman, and Geoffrey L. Cohen, "Self-Affirmation Facilitates Minority Middle Schoolers' Progress Along College Trajectories," *Proceedings of the National Academy of Sciences* 114, no. 29 (2017): 7594–99, https://doi.org/10.1073/pnas.1617923114.

190 *examine cultural trends in the United States*: Pelin Kesebir and Selin Kesebir, "The Cultural Salience of Moral Character and Virtue Decline in Twentieth Century America," *Journal of Positive Psychology* 7, no. 6 (2012): 471–80.

198 *A study of nearly 4,000 US military veterans*: Hun Kang, Ian C. Fischer, Samuel Dickinson, Peter J. Na, Jack Tsai, Richard G. Tedeschi, and Robert H. Pietrzak, "Posttraumatic Growth in U.S. Military Veterans: Results from the National Health and Resilience in Veterans Study," *Psychiatric Quarterly* 95, no. 1 (2024): 17–32, https://doi.org/10.1007/s11126-023-10061-8.

198 *higher levels of purpose were linked to lower levels of PTSD symptoms*: Adriana Feder, Samoon Ahmad, Elisa J. Lee, Julia E. Morgan, Ritika Singh, Bruce W. Smith, Steven M. Southwick, and Dennis S. Charney, "Coping and PTSD Symptoms in Pakistani Earthquake Survivors: Purpose in Life, Religious Coping and Social Support," *Journal of Affective Disorders* 147, no. 1–3 (2013): 156–63, https://doi.org/10.1016/j.jad.2012.10.027. For a review and meta-analysis of this literature, see Maryam Hosseinnejad, Vahid Yazdi-Feyzabadi, Ahmad Hajebi, Ali Bahramnejad, Reza Baneshi, Roghayeh Ershad Sarabi, Maryam Okhovati, Razieh Zahedi, Hossein Saberi, and Farzaneh Zolala, "Prevalence of Posttraumatic Stress Disorder Following the Earthquake in Iran and Pakistan: A Systematic Review and Meta-Analysis," *Disaster Medicine and Public Health Preparedness* 16, no. 2 (2022): 801–8, https://doi.org/10.1017/dmp.2020.411.

198 *Scientists have observed that some cancer patients seem to undergo a profound personal transformation*: Lyndel K. Shand, Sean Cowlishaw, Joanne E. Brooker, Sue Burney, and Lina A. Ricciardelli, "Correlates of Post-Traumatic Stress Symptoms and Growth in Cancer Patients: A Systematic Review and Meta-Analysis," *Psycho-Oncology* 24, no. 6 (2015): 624–34, https://doi.org/10.1002/pon.3719. For a review, see: Allison Marziliano, Malwina Tuman, and Anne Moyer, "The Relationship Between Post-Traumatic Stress and Post-Traumatic Growth in Cancer Patients and Survivors: A Systematic Review and Meta-Analysis," *Psycho-Oncology* 29, no. 4 (2020): 604–16, https://doi.org/10.1002/pon.5314.

199 *An inspiring example of this comes from Viktor Frankl's* Man's Search for Meaning: Viktor E. Frankl, *Man's Search for Meaning* (Boston: Beacon Press, 2006).

Chapter 9: Making Flourishing a Habit

213 *The article featured three people*: Malcolm Gladwell, "The Physical Genius," *New Yorker*, July 25, 1999.

213 *Practicing for five minutes a day for thirty days is of greater benefit*: M. J. Hirshberg, C. Frye, C. J. Dahl, K. M. Riordan, N. J. Vack, J. Sachs, R. Goldman, R. J. Davidson, and S. B. Goldberg, "A Randomized Controlled Trial of a Smartphone-Based Well-Being Training in Public School System Employees During the COVID-19 Pandemic," *Journal of Educational Psychology* 114, no. 8 (2022): 1895–1911, https://doi.org/10.1037/edu0000739.

214 *In science, we call the zeitgeber a "circadian time cue"*: Cindy L. Ehlers, Ellen Frank, and David J. Kupfer, "Social Zeitgebers and Biological Rhythms: A Unified Approach to Understanding the Etiology of Depression," *Archives of General Psychiatry* 45, no. 10 (1988): 948–52, https://doi: 10.1001/archpsyc.1988.01800340076012.

Chapter 10: Change Your Mind, Change the World

223 *The employees of the Louisville school system became more welcoming*: Matthew J. Hirshberg et al., "Enhancing Student Math Achievement Through a Digital Wellbeing Training for Educators" (2025), under review.

223 *worked with this school for five years, bringing simple flourishing practices*: Ilana Shlomov, Nava Levit-Binnun, and Tzipi Horowitz-Kraus, "Neurodevelopmental Effects of a Mindfulness and Kindness Curriculum on Executive Functions in Preschool Children—A Randomized, Active-Controlled Study," *Mind, Brain, and Education* 17, no. 2 (2023): 132–48, https://doi.org/10.1111/mbe.12348.

224 *We know that having a strong sense of purpose is the most important psychological predictor of longevity among people 70 years of age and older*: This is a classic study that first showed this in a large sample: Patrick L. Hill and Nicholas A. Turiano, "Purpose in Life as a Predictor of Mortality Across Adulthood," *Psychological Science* 25, no. 7 (2014): 1482–86, https://doi.org/10.1177/0956797614531799. This

is a study that nicely establishes that it is purpose in life rather than other related psychological constructs that most strongly predicts longevity: Frank Martela, Elmeri Laitinen, and Christian Hakulinen, "Which Predicts Longevity Better: Satisfaction with Life or Purpose in Life?" *Psychology and Aging* 39 (2024): 589–98, https://doi.org/10.1037/pag0000802.supp.

225 *Research by the Johns Hopkins group shows*: Michelle C. Carlson, Kirk I. Erickson, Arthur F. Kramer, Michelle W. Voss, Natalie Bolea, Michelle Mielke, Sylvia McGill, George W. Rebok, Teresa Seeman, and Linda P. Fried, "Evidence for Neurocognitive Plasticity in At-Risk Older Adults: The Experience Corps Program," *The Journals of Gerontology Series A, Biological Sciences and Medical Sciences* 64, no. 12 (2009): 1275–82, https://doi.org/10.1093/gerona/glp117.

Index

AARP, 226
abused children, 58–60
action(s)
    in developing habits, 211–13
    disconnect between beliefs and, 181
    dysfunctional, 84
    small, 23
    see also behaviors
active meditations, 17
    Commuting with Connection, 245
    Finding Meaning in the Mundane, 254–55
    Morning Routine with Awareness, 239–40
    Thoughts Shape Reality, 250
adaptability, flourishing as, 16
adaptation, in the body, 28
addiction
    current crisis in, 18
    to smartphones, 47–48
adversity
    changing relationship to, 27 (*see also* challenges)
    early experiences of, 58–60
    finding purpose in, 185–87
    flourishing in the face of, 63–65
    inner narrative about, 157
    learning in midst of, 69
    reframing, 200
    trauma as subjective interpretation of, 59
advertising, fear-based, 26–27
affection, 123
affordances, 206
aging, sense of purpose in, 184, 224–26
aloneness
    in a crowd, 126–27
    on work video calls, 131
    see also loneliness

altruism, 14
    acts of, 210
    brain activity patterns linked to, 143–44
    Dalai Lama on mindset for, 85–86
    and innate goodness, 36–40
    multiplicative benefits of, 226
"Altruism and Compassion in Economic Systems," 6
Alzheimer's disease, 33, 36
amygdala, 27
    brain regions connected to, 28
    and early-life trauma, 59
    salience network in activation of, 107
    in threat detection, 54
analytical meditation
    to cultivate wisdom, 80
    Dalai Lama on, 173
    as path to insight, 166
anger
    and connection, 124
    given the state of the world, 220
anxiety(-ies)
    bodily feelings of, 23
    causes of, 45–47
    current age of, 118–19
    and exposure to the news, 54
    and feeling of connection, 127
    five-minute daily practice for reducing, 13
    heritability of, 61–63
    inner narrative about, 164
    as outcome of evolutionary wiring, 45–46
    seeds of flourishing in, 24
    and smartphone addiction, 48
    social, 53
apathy
    and connection, 124
    transforming, 145

Index

appreciation, 27
    cultivating, 92
    extending feelings of, 83
    feelings of connection with, 124, 125, 130
    generating feelings of, 133–37
    Morning Moments of, 41
    noticing and nurturing moments of, 132
    in strengthening connection, 82
    tempering grief with, 128
    for yourself, 138
Aristotle, 69, 203
artistic traditions, awareness-based, 115
assumptions
    examining, 154–55
    insight into, 152
    seeing beyond your, 84
    shifting to curiosity from, 148 (*see also* insight)
asthma, 36
attention
    of advanced meditators, 75, 78, 104
    in awareness practices, 112–13
    and brain networks, 87, 104
    and distractions, 48–50
    as element of awareness, 102, 103
    feelings in moments of, 24
    mastery of, 78
    for mental health and emotional well-being, 87
    as quality of flourishing, 73
    research on, 7–8
    in social interactions, 115–16
    training, 82
    see also focus
auditory cortex, 27–28
authenticity
    in connection, 185
    by the Dalai Lama, 123
    in transformation, 221
automatic thoughts, 159–60
autonomy, as dimension of well-being, 184
awareness, 8, 97–119
    of advanced meditators, 75–76
    being in touch with, 102
    brain changes from, 27
    and brain networks, 15, 104, 106–8
    building practice of, 111–15
    as central to mental health and emotional well-being, 87
    combination of connection, insight, and, 78–79, 174
    connecting with, 105
    cultivating, 104, 115–16
    defined, 10, 102
    described, 101–3
    of distractions, 49
    and experiential fusion, 108, 109
    of feelings, 22
    five-minute daily practice for, 13
    and flow, 110–11
    Healthy Minds Meditation for, 235–36
    linking daily activities to, 206
    main benefits of, 105–6
    measuring, 88–90
    meta-awareness, 108–9
    mindfulness vs., 108
    mind's untapped potential for, 119
    of Mingyur Rinpoche, 76
    movement from distraction to, 108
    in observing inner narrative, 164
    open, 79–80, 113–15
    in path to flourishing, 82
    power of, 100–101
    practices for, 13, 17, 82, 103, 111–15, 235–42
    as prerequisite for change, 46–47
    present-moment, 99–100
    "pure awareness," 80, 171
    recognizing presence of, 70
    research on, 11
    rewiring brain with, 117–18
    as a skill, 104–6
    spillover effect of, 117
    strengthening, 92
    and theories of well-being, 86–87
    of values, 192
    world's need for, 118–19
    in world's wisdom traditions, 81
awareness-based meditation, brain change from, 30–32

balance
    in challenging circumstances, 45
    daily rituals for living with, 15
    helping others nurture, 222
    in holding beliefs, 161–63
    of salience and executive networks, 107–8
Beck, Aaron, 153
behavioral changes
    building conscious habits for, 206–8
    due to social isolation, 52–53
    learning to make, 12
    toward flourishing, 55

Index

behaviors
    habits as (*see* habits [in general])
    heritability of, 61–63
    unhealthy, perpetuation of, 150
being, shift from doing to, 113–15
beliefs
    disconnect between actions and, 181
    examining, 153–55
    experiences shaped by, 25
    healthy way of holding, 161–63
    insight into, 152
    letting go of, 84
    in life of purpose and meaning, 184
    limiting, 150
    in our inner narrative, 148
    rumination fueled by, 159
    that shape experience, 148
    unhealthy emotional habits and thought patterns created by, 85
"benefiting all beings," Tibetans' commitment to, 177–78
biases, in inner narratives, 157
bodhichitta, 79
body
    change and adaptation in, 28–29
    mind-brain-body interaction, 53
    pliability/plasticity of, 25–32
    training of, 80–81
    understanding sensations in, 23–24
    see also physical health
Boudhanath, Kathmandu, 175–76
Boudhanath stupa, 36–37, 176
brain(s)
    of advanced meditators vs. non-meditators, 71, 74–78, 117
    in anxious rats study, 62–63
    awareness affecting networks of, 104, 106–8
    changed by experience and training, 30–32
    effect of early trauma on, 58–60
    gamma activity in, 170–71
    insight's effect on, 155–58
    of "masters of insight," 169–72
    during meditation, 75
    of meditators, 12–13
    mind-brain-body interaction, 53
    networks underlying connection in, 141–44
    neuroplasticity of, 25–32, 60 (*see also* rewiring the brain)
    pathways between body and, 28–32
    in resting state, 117
    and smartphone addiction, 47–48
    social isolation's effect on, 52–53
    threat circuitry in, 54–55
    see also specific brain structures and networks
brain waves, 170
Buber, Martin, 212
Buddhism
    Dalai Lama on using practices of, 173
    in Nepal, 175
    see also Tibetan Buddhism
burnout, 220

Calendar, Compassionate, 140–41
calligraphy, 115
calm
    with awareness, 119
    neural impulses with, 29
    from practicing awareness, 117
cancer, flourishing program's effect on, 60
cardiovascular disease
    flourishing program's effect on, 60
    inflammation component of, 36
care network (in brain), 132, 142–43
caring
    among Tibetan refugees, 178
    in cultural analysis, 191
    by the Dalai Lama, 123, 124
    driven by compassion, 125
    generating emotions/feelings of, 83–84, 133, 134
    helped by insight, 150
    of Mingyur Rinpoche, 76
    for people or groups we dislike, 137–38
    as quality of flourishing, 73
caring listening, flourishing as, 16
Center for Healthy Minds (CHM), 4, 6, 7, 258
    awareness research at, 31–32, 46–47, 104, 117–18
    benefits from program of, 13
    epigenetic research at, 34–36
    flourishing cities, 228–29
    meditation training research of, 160–61
    remote workers at, 52
    and repetition in establishing habits, 213
    trauma research at, 58–59
Center for Mindfulness in Medicine, Health Care, and Society, 111
central executive network, 106
certainty, shifting to open-mindedness from, 148

Index

challenge(s), 43–65
    applying habits for flourishing amid, 216–17
    being transformed by, 23–24, 45
    brain and body changes from, 27–28
    and causes of anxiety, overwhelm, and depression, 45–47
    developing different relationship with, 23
    digital world as, 47–48
    distraction as, 48–51
    finding purpose in, 194–95
    flourishing amid, 8, 16, 53–54, 63–65, 179–80
    genetics as, 60–63
    insight from reflection on, 150
    money as, 55–58
    as opportunities for self-exploration, 23
    post-traumatic growth from, 197–99
    presence and awareness in, 100–101
    resilience as response to, 5
    social isolation as, 52–53
    transformed by sense of purpose, 187
    trauma as, 58–60
    twenty-four-hour news cycle as, 54–55
    see also adversity
change, 219–29
    awareness as prerequisite for, 46–47
    in the body, 25–32
    in the brain, 25–32 (*see also* rewiring the brain)
    to build flourishing cities, 228–29
    building conscious habits for, 206–8
    epigenetics and potential for, 32–36
    in experience of pain, 221–22
    finding individual recipes for, 226–27
    from insight, 152
    and need for purpose, 224–26
    in people practicing Tibetan Buddhism, 70–71
    positive vs. negative, 25–26
    in problems facing the world, 219–21
    Sitting Meditation–Opening to Change, 247–49
    widening effect of flourishing for, 222–24
children, abused/maltreated, 58–60
CHM, *see* Center for Healthy Minds
choiceless awareness practice, 113
choices
    insight practices giving different set of, 165
    small, growth through, 24
    see also action(s); behaviors
chronic illnesses, 36

chronic stress, 45
    beliefs leading to, 85
    from overactive threat response, 151
    triggered by default-mode network, 158
circadian rhythms
    gene expression affected by, 34
    habits added to natural time cues, 214–15
cities, flourishing, 228–29
climate crisis, 221
closed-mindedness, 161–63
cognitive function/abilities, sense of purpose and, 184, 200
cognitive insight, 153
cognitive reappraisal, 143, 144, 160
Collins, Francis, 121, 122
commitment
    to flourishing, 15
    intention as, 210
communication
    of deepest values, 185
    flourishing skills transforming, 161–63
    Insight Through Dialogue, 168–69
    reflective dialogue, 167
    see also listening
communities, flourishing in, 222–23
compassion, 5
    brain circuits underlying, 14
    combined with insight and self-knowledge, 171
    of the Dalai Lama, 123, 124
    Dalai Lama on, 173
    extending feelings of, 83
    feelings of connection with, 124, 125
    generating, 83–84, 133, 134
    and innate goodness, 36–40
    journaling to nurture, 139
    in observing inner narrative, 164
    practicing, 14, 15, 216–17
    relationship of empathy and, 142–43
    research on, 7–8
    in strengthening connection, 82–83
    of Tibetan monks, 72
    Writing Reflection–Remembering Compassion, 246
    for yourself, 138
Compassionate Calendar, 140–41
competing demands, 23
concentration, 75–78
concentration impairments, 5
connection, 8, 121–45
    by advanced meditators, 75–76
    with all forms of life, 78–79

Index

with awareness, 105
brain networks underlying, 141–44
brain's pain network changed by, 15
building practice of, 131–33
combination of awareness, insight, and, 78–79, 174
creating cues for, 212
defined, 10, 124
feelings of, 124–28
five-minute daily practice for, 13
flourishing as, 16, 25
formal and informal practices for, 93
Healthy Minds Meditation for, 235–36
heartwarming, 24
and innate goodness, 36–40
limitless potential for, 145
measuring, 88–90
nurturing moments of, 131–32
objective vs. subjective, 126–27
and observation of inner narrative, 164
in path to flourishing, 82–84
power of, 123–24
practices for, 13, 17, 82–84, 93, 129, 131–41, 235–36, 242–47
recognizing patterns of, 185
research on, 11
resulting from attention, 3
ruined by distraction, 50
self-transcendence as, 152
as a skill, 130–31
and smartphone use, 48
and social isolation, 52–53
in theories of well-being, 86
through deep conversations, 23
Tibetan spiritual practices of, 74
in time of loss or grief, 64–65
widening circle of, 83, 136–38
in world's wisdom traditions, 81
see also social interactions
conscious habits
adding zeitgebers to, 214–15
developing, 205–8
see also habits for flourishing; routines
consciousness
discovering more subtle dimensions of, 150
forms of meditation exploring, 80
insight into nature of, 78–79
nature and transformation of, 75, 171
as quality of the mind, 101
contemplative practice, 7–8
dimensions of flourishing in, 81

in Healthy Minds Program, 174
insight produced by, 85
rewiring brain through, 13
see also meditation
context, connection to, 25
cortisol, 34
courage, 45, 187
Covid-19 pandemic
feelings of connection during, 127
remote work following, 52
as time of extreme stress, 13
creativity
and brain networks, 158
flourishing as, 16
Csikszentmihalyi, Mihaly, 110
cues, 212
in forming habits, 205–6 (*see also* habits for flourishing)
natural/circadian time cues, 214–15
as reminders of skills, 226, 227
cultures, analyzing, 190–91
curiosity
about your beliefs, 162–63
about your habits and reactions, 151
about your mind, 152
in developing insight, 84, 159–61
in self-inquiry, 159
shifting from assumptions to, 148 (*see also* insight)

daily life
applying purpose in, 193–94
awareness in, 105, 116
developing conscious habits in, 205–8
distraction in, 48–50
extending purpose in, 194–95
and impact of what you feed your mind on, 190–91
informal practice in, 93
knowing your purpose in, 181
making time for skills practice in, 226–27
practicing flourishing in activities of, 91–92
rushed activity in, 176–77
daily meditation practice, 80–81
daily rituals
to calm mind and live with balance, 15
in creating habits for flourishing (*see* habits for flourishing)
to nurture the best in self, 191–92
see also practices for flourishing; routines

Index

Dalai Lama, 6
    ability to connect by, 123–24
    advice and encouragement from, 5–6
    authenticity of, 123
    briefings on scientific advances for, 61
    flourishing skills practiced by, 209
    at inauguration of Center for Healthy Minds, 4
    on insight, 172–73
    on kindness, 121
    National Institutes of Health visit by, 121–23
    on practice for altruistic mindset, 85–86
    practice of, 133
    Ronan's meeting with, 221
    Tibet fled by, 175
Danese, Andrea, 59
"deaths of despair," 46
Deaton, Angus, 46
decentering, 163, 165
declarative-procedural gap, 12
default-mode network
    connection between executive network and, 160–61
    and distraction, 117
    and inner narration, 158
    and self-regulation, 118
delta waves, 170
dementia, 36
depression, 4, 5
    and ability to grow new neurons, 32
    causes of, 45–47
    current crisis in, 18
    and exposure to the news, 54
    and feeling of connection, 127
    five-minute daily practice to improve, 13
    as outcome of evolutionary wiring, 45–46
    resilience as response to, 5
    seeds of flourishing in, 24
    and smartphone addiction, 48
de-reification, 164
despair, given state of the world, 220
dialogue
    Insight Through, 168–69
    reflective, 167
didactic learning, 12
difficulties, *see* challenges
digital devices
    challenge with, 47–48
    creating connection when relating through, 130–31
    as distraction, 48–50

direction, sense of, 184
discipline, in remaining curious, 161
disconnection, noticing moments of, 131–32
disease/illness
    flourishing through, 43–45
    genes for, 33
    inflammation component of, 36
    see also individual conditions
distal outcomes, 228–29
distortions, in inner narratives, 157, 165
distractibility, 5, 18
distraction
    advanced meditators' resistance to, 77–78
    brain regions linked to, 117
    cost of, 48–51
    current age of, 118–19
    as major obstacle to flourishing, 41
    mind-wandering as, 117
    movement to awareness from, 108
    seeds of flourishing in, 24
    stress resulting from, 105
Distraction Reflection, 51
distress, empathic, 142
DNA methylation, 35
doing, shift to being from, 113–15
doomscrolling, 26, 50, 150
dorsolateral prefrontal cortex, 118, 144
doubts, rumination fueled by, 159
dreaming, 77
dream yoga, 77
Dzogchen, 80, 171

ease, feelings in moments of, 24
eating, conscious, 214–15
economic growth, well-being vs., 55
Emerson, Ralph Waldo, 3
emotional habits
    beliefs creating, 85
    insight into, 150, 152
emotional health
    conscious regulation of, 106
    flourishing skills' role in, 86
emotional reactions/reactivity
    decentering in observation of, 164
    defusing, 159
    self-regulation of, 160
emotional resilience, 184
emotional responses
    of advanced meditators, 75
    meta-awareness of, 109
    and salience network, 107

Index

emotional well-being
    caring relationships and interactions shaping, 125–26
    in challenging situations, 56–57
    feelings of connection affecting, 127
emotions
    awareness in managing, 106
    being present to your, 112
    body and brain traces of, 29
    bringing awareness to, 22–24
    in connection, 124–28 (*see also* connection)
    curiosity and self-inquiry about, 160
    de-reification of, 164
    developing insight through, 84
    feeling in control of, 17
    gene expression influenced by, 33–34
    insight into, 8, 150
    managing vs. being ruled by, 149
    as perception of bodily change, 28–29
    positive, five-minute daily practice for, 13
    science of, 7–8
    from social comparison, defusing, 58
    as "soft skills," 142
    in tempering grief, 128
    that shape experience, 148
    see also specific emotions
empathic distress, 142
empathy
    brain regions linked to, 144
    flourishing as, 16
    helped by insight, 150
    relationship of compassion and, 142–43
    research on, 7–8
environment, in anxious rats study, 62–63
environmental mastery, as dimension of well-being, 184
epigenetics, 25–26, 32–36
    altered by mental training, 34–36
    changed by flourishing program, 60
    changes in response to experience, 61–63
    defined, 25
    factors in extent of gene expression, 33
    of stress, 34
epiphanies, 152
equanimity, research on, 7–8
eudaimonic well-being, 69
everyday life, *see* daily life
executive network
    and awareness, 106–8
    in compassion training, 144
    connection between default-mode network and, 160–61
    default-mode network modulation by, 158
expectations
    experiences shaped by, 25
    seeing beyond your, 84
Experience Corps, 225–26
experience(s)
    biology altered by, 61–62
    brain links between different modes of, 67
    of early trauma, 58–60
    experiential fusion vs. meta-awareness in, 109
    flexible attentiveness to, 103
    of flow, 110–11
    heightened attentiveness to, 102–3
    inner narratives in making sense of, 157
    interneuron growth and change from, 30
    "I-Thou," 212
    learning and growth from, 156
    linking acts of curiosity to, 161
    of pain, 97–100, 221–22
    self-inquiry for insights into, 159
    subjective, 59–60
    that bring out our very best, 45 (*see also* challenge[s])
    thoughts, emotions, and beliefs shaping, 148 (*see also* insight)
    transcendent, 152–53
experience sampling, 49
experiential fusion, 108, 109
Extinction Rebellion, 221

failed relationships, 185
fear
    and connection, 124
    and loneliness, 53
    seeds of flourishing in, 24
    US election advertising based on, 25–27
feeling connected, 124–28
    see also connection
fight-flight-freeze response, 29, 151
financial health, sense of purpose for, 184
flexible attentiveness, 103
flourishing, 3–19
    all of life affected by, 189
    amid challenges/hardships, 63–65, 69
    community and individual, 222–23
    constraints on, 47
    core dimensions of, 25, 81–86

Index

flourishing (cont.)
    cultivating (see path to flourishing)
    despite challenges, 53–54
    distal outcomes of, 228–29
    embodying qualities of, 229
    framework for, 86–90 (see also Healthy Minds Framework)
    genetic factors in, 60–63
    growth of new neurons for, 32
    happiness vs., 16–18, 63
    innate capacities for, 40, 220–21
    intergenerationally transmitted qualities of, 35
    learning of, 76
    and mindfulness practice, 7–9
    moments of, 3–4
    nature of, 69
    as practice, not destination, 24
    practices for, 12–15 (see also practices for flourishing)
    pre-wiring for, 55
    and procedural vs. didactic learning, 12
    realistic possibility of, 53–54
    scientific models of, 70
    skills of, 8, 10–11, 16 (see also skills for flourishing)
    through illness, 43–45
    and tipping point for humanity, 5–7
    widening effect of, 222–24
flourishing cities, 228–29
flow, awareness and, 110–11
flower arrangement, awareness-based, 115
focus
    with awareness, 119
    and executive network, 106
    feelings in moments of, 24
    five-minute daily practice to improve, 13
    flourishing as, 16
    of Mingyur Rinpoche, 76, 77
    rewiring brain for, 4
    in social situations, 116
formal practices, 92–94
Frankl, Viktor, 199
frustration, 136

gamma oscillations, 11, 170–71
Gandhi, Mahatma, 43
gene expression, 25–26, 32–36
    see also epigenetics
generosity, 37
    engaging in, 210
    of Tibetan refugees, 178

genetics
    as challenge to flourishing, 60–63
    in exclusion of others, 83
    tapping potential of, 78
    see also epigenetics
Gilbert, Dan, 49, 50
Gladwell, Malcolm, 213
global crises and upheaval, 118–19, 219
goals, meaningful, 184
Goldsmith, Hill, 38–39
goodness, innate, 36–40
goodwill, expressing feelings of, 134–35
gratitude
    creating cues for, 212
    research on, 7–8
    tempering grief with, 128
gratitude journaling, 83–84
Gretzky, Wayne, 213
grief
    experiencing love and connection during, 64–65
    from failed relationships, 185
    tempered with nourishing emotions, 128
growth
    amid adversity, 185–86, 187
    capitalist society orientation toward, 55
    in challenging situations, 180
    as dimension of well-being, 184
    from experiences, 156
    insight as catalyst for, 149
    Journaling Reflection–Opportunities for Growth, 240–41
    post-traumatic, 197–99
    transforming challenge into, 24
    Writing Reflection–What Leads to Growth and Insight?, 251

habits (in general)
    acting out of awareness instead of, 101
    conscious, 205, 211
    curiosity about, 151, 159
    in distracted driving, 105–6
    of distraction, 51
    emotional, beliefs creating, 85
    establishing, 217
    executive network in breaking and building, 106
    healthy, 204
    mental, 164
    opportunities for creating, 216–17
    positive vs. negative, 26

short-circuited by openness and curiosity, 160
  steps in creating, 208–14
habits for flourishing, 203–17
  action, 211–13
  added to natural time cues, 214–15
  applied amid challenges, 216–17
  brain and body changes with, 32
  conscious, 205–8
  in daily life, 15
  daily meditation practice, 80–81
  establishing, 217
  innate capacity to develop, 9
  inspiration, 208–10
  intention, 40, 210–11
  procedural learning in establishing, 12
  repetition, 213–14
  in reversing mental health decline, 14–15
  steps in developing, 208–14
Hamlin, Kiley, 39
Hanson, Jamie, 58–59
happiness
  assumption that money equals, 55
  from benefiting all beings, 177
  flourishing vs., 16–18, 63
  Keller on, 85
  learning, 76
  when distracted, 49–50
hardships
  relieving, 125 (*see also* compassion)
  see also challenge(s)
Harrington, Ronan, 221, 222
hatha yoga, 115
healing power of connection, 123
health, *see* mental health; physical health
Health Enhancement Program, 31, 118
Healthy Minds Framework, 10, 16
  basis for, 79
  development of, 86–90 (*see also* path to flourishing)
  example of, 16–18
  insight in, 172–73
  origin of, 87
Healthy Minds Index, 88–91
Healthy Minds Innovations (HMI), *see* Humin
"Healthy Minds Meditation, The," 93–94
Healthy Minds Program, 258
  app for, 17, 18
  contemplative practices and science in, 174
  in improving a marriage, 151

heartwarming connection, 24
hedonic well-being, 69
heightened attentiveness, 102
helping others, 177, 220
heritability studies, 60–63
hierarchy of needs, 56
hippocampus, 30, 59
Hirshberg, Matt, 127

Holocaust survivors, 34, 199
humanity
  Dalai Lama on, 221
  factors supporting or limiting flourishing for, 45–46
  future of, 229
  tipping point for, 5–7
Humin, 4, 17, 232, 259
humor, of Tibetan monks, 72

identity
  created with memories and thoughts, 150
  in times of adversity, 186–87
illness, *see* disease/illness
imagination
  harnessing power of, 158
  see also creativity; curiosity
impulses
  awareness in managing, 106
  as driver when distracted, 105–6
  insight into, 150
  and salience network, 107
income inequality, perceived, 57
income satiation, 56–57
inflammation
  decreased with meditation, 25
  flourishing program's effect on, 60
  gene activation for, 33
  in meditators, 35–36
  and sleep-wake transitions, 34
inflammatory bowel disease, 36
informal practices, 92–94
innate capacities for flourishing, 40, 220–21
innate goodness, 36–40
inner mastery
  of advanced meditators, 72, 76, 171–72
  of Mingyur Rinpoche, 77
inner narratives, 68, 148, 149
  and brain's default-mode network, 158
  in making sense of experiences, 157
  transforming, 164–65
inner peace, as quality of flourishing, 73

insight, 147–74
    brain affected by, 15, 155–58
    brains of "masters of insight," 169–72
    cognitive, 153
    combination of awareness, connection, and, 78–79, 174
    combined with compassion and self-knowledge, 171
    cultivating, 92, 172–74
    and curiosity, 159–61
    defined, 11, 149
    formal and informal practices for, 93
    Healthy Minds Meditation for, 235–36
    and healthy way of holding beliefs, 161–63
    and inner narrative, 164–65
    from life challenges, 45
    measuring, 88–90
    into nature of consciousness, 78–79
    and pain network, 15
    in path to flourishing, 84–85
    pathways to, 166–67
    power of, 149–53
    practices for, 13, 17, 84–85, 154–55, 168–69, 235–36, 247–52
    as quality of flourishing, 73
    recognizing and celebrating, 156
    research on, 11
    and theories of well-being, 86–87
    into thoughts and emotions, 8
    Tibetan spiritual practices of, 74
    in world's wisdom traditions, 81
Insight Through Dialogue, 168–69
inspiration, in developing habits, 208–10
insula, 28, 53
intention
    in awareness practices, 111–12
    to be kind, 137
    decentering thoughts for, 165
    in developing habits, 210–11
    in engaging with the world, 27
    for formal practice, 92–93
    infusing routines with, 204
    in practice for flourishing, 91, 92
    in remaining curious, 161
    in rewiring the brain, 40
    in smartphone use, 50
    in social interactions, 115–16
interneurons, 29–39
Interpersonal Practice
    Exploring the Web of Causes and Conditions, 252

Listening with Mindful Awareness, 241–42
100th Birthday Party, 257
Warm Memories, 247
interpretation(s)
    in the brain, 156
    faulty, seeing through, 149 (*see also* insight)
    subjective, of adversity, 59
    through inner narrative, 157
"I-Thou" experiences, 212

James, LeBron, 56
James, William, 28
Johns Hopkins University, 225–26
journaling
    for connection, 134
    gratitude, 83–84
    insight from, 150
    to nurture kindness and compassion, 139
    to reframe current challenge, 196–97
    see also reflective writing
Journaling Reflection–Opportunities for Growth, 240–41
joy
    in Boudhanath, 176
    human preference for, 37
    of Tibetan monks, 72
Joy of Living, The (Mingyur Rinpoche), 76
judgments
    in inner narratives, 157
    rumination fueled by, 159
Jung, Carl, 21

Kabat-Zinn, Jon, 111, 118
Kaliman, Perla, 35
Kathmandu, Nepal, 175–76
Keller, Helen, 85
Kesebir, Pelin, 190–91
Kesebir, Selin, 190–91
Killingsworth, Matt, 49, 50
kindness
    brain circuits underlying, 14
    in cultural analysis, 191
    of the Dalai Lama, 124
    Dalai Lama on, 121
    extending feelings of, 83
    feelings of connection with, 124, 125
    generating feelings of, 133, 134
    and innate goodness, 36–40
    journaling to nurture, 139
    learning, 12

of Mingyur Rinpoche, 76
noticing and nurturing moments of, 132
in observing inner narrative, 164
for people or groups we dislike, 137–38
research on, 7–8
setting an intention for, 137
Sitting Meditation–Extending Kindness in New Directions, 242–44
in strengthening connection, 82
of Tibetan refugees, 178
Kral, Tammi, 31–32

land, relationship to, 220
learning
    action in, 211–13
    in adversity, 69, 185
    in the brain, 156
    to flourish, 4, 9, 12–15, 76
    humans' ability for, 30
    inspiration in, 208–10
    intention in, 210–11
    procedural vs. didactic, 12
    repetition in, 213–14
    steps involved in, 208
    through osmosis, 229
Levit-Binnun, Nava, 223, 224
life circumstances
    gene expression influenced by, 33–34
    that bring out our very best, 45 (*see also* challenge[s])
    see also daily life
life expectancy, 18
    in developed countries, 46
    increase in, 224–25
    in the United States, 5
life satisfaction, exposure to the news and, 54
limiting beliefs, 150
listening
    awareness in, 119
    caring listening, flourishing as, 16
    Interpersonal Practice–Listening with Mindful Awareness, 241–42
    power of, 23
    when your beliefs are challenged, 162–63
loneliness, 4
    current crisis of, 18
    as danger to health, 5
    decreasing, 127–28
    as premature mortality risk factor, 52
    and social isolation, 52–53
loss, experiencing love and connection during, 64–65

Louisville, Kentucky school system, 222–23
love
    of the Dalai Lama, 123
    as essential relationship ingredient, 44–45
    generating, 83–84
    in time of loss or grief, 64–65
loving-kindness meditations, 84
luminosity meditation, 77
Lutz, Antoine, 35, 97, 98

Ma, Yo-Yo, 213
Mahamudra, 69–70, 80
Malaktaris, Anne, 15
Mandela, Nelson, 179–80, 197
Man's Search for Meaning (Frankl), 199
Marcus Aurelius, 115
martial arts, 115
Maslow, Abraham, 55–56
Max Planck Institute, 160
MBSR (Mindfulness-Based Stress Reduction) Program, 118
Meaney, Michael, 61–63
meaning, 8
    Active Meditation–Finding Meaning in the Mundane, 254–55
    brought by sense of purpose, 177 (*see also* purpose)
    in cultural analysis, 191
    and emotional balance, 11
    five-minute daily practice for, 13
    found in the mundane, 187–89
    pursuit of, 69
    and salience network, 29
meaningful life
    building a, 199–200
    mundane moments vs., 179
    purpose in, 177, 184
meaningful moments, in mundane moments, 183, 187–89
measuring skills of flourishing, 88–90
meditation, 4
    active, 17
    analytical, 166, 173
    awareness-based, 30–32
    brain rewired by, 12–13, 71, 74–78, 117
    brain's pain network changed by, 15
    compassion practice, 14, 15
    to cultivate wisdom, 80
    Dzogchen, 80
    epigenetic change from, 25, 35–36
    establishing daily practice of, 217
    gamma oscillations during, 11

Index

meditation (*cont.*)
    with Healthy Minds Program app, 18
    insight, 17
    loving-kindness, 84
    Mahamudra, 69–70, 80
    mindfulness, 44, 79
    Mingyur Rinpoche's practices of, 79–80
    NIH funding for research on, 121
    "Olympian" meditator studies, 104, 169–70
    open awareness, 113–15
    outlook changed by, 64
    and pain response, 97–100
    power of, 5
    research on, 104
    research on practitioners of, 6, 74–76 (*see also* path to flourishing)
    Shamatha, 173
    in strengthening connection, 82–83
    see also practices for flourishing; *specific meditations*
memory(-ies)
    of emotions, 29
    hippocampus's role in, 30
    Interpersonal Practice–Warm Memories, 247
    meaningful, purpose discovered in, 193
    painful, 161
    sense of identity created with, 150
    Sitting Meditation–Meaningful Memories, 252–54
    and visualization, 67
mental health
    caring relationships and interactions shaping, 125–26
    connection for, 129
    conscious regulation of, 106
    current crisis in, 5, 18, 52
    and default-mode network, 158
    eroded by worry and stress, 46
    feelings of connection affecting, 127
    five-minute daily practice to improve, 13
    flourishing skills in reversing decline of, 14–15
    flourishing skills' role in, 86
    mindfulness practice alone for, 7
    reversing current trends around, 9, 10
    sabotaged by inner narratives, 157
    scientific models of, 104
    sense of purpose for, 184
    and sleep-wake transitions, 34
    and smartphone addiction, 48
    and subjective report of trauma, 59
    toll of chronic stress on, 151
mental illness, cognitive insight into, 153
meta-awareness, 108–12
micro-supports
    in flourishing cities, 228
    for habits, 215
mind
    awareness of what is happening in, 109
    curiosity about your, 152
    in experience of pain, 15
    insight into your, 84
    Mahamudra in exploring and transforming, 70
    mind-brain-body interaction, 53
    narratives/stories constructed in (*see* inner narratives)
    nourishing your, 190–92
    quality of consciousness in, 101
    rumination by, 159
    shift toward flourishing in, 55 (*see also* path to flourishing)
    stress levels of, 118–19
    training, 27, 79–81 (*see also* rewiring the brain)
    unhealthy states of, 32
    untapped potential of, 119
    wandering, 31–32, 50, 117, 160
    see also thoughts
mind-brain-body interaction, 53
mindful awareness, 78
    to direct attention and regulate mind-wandering, 31–32
    Interpersonal Practice–Listening with Mindful Awareness, 241–42
    practicing awareness vs., 111
mindfulness
    awareness vs., 108
    classes for, 115
    Dalai Lama on, 172–73
    defined, 108, 111
    five-minute daily practice to improve, 13
    flourishing vs., 7–9
    as only one form of meditation, 79
    research on, 87, 104
Mindfulness-Based Stress Reduction (MBSR) Program, 118
Mindfulness-Based Stress Reduction Clinic, 111
mindfulness meditation, 44, 79
Mind & Life Institute, 6

Index

Mingyur Rinpoche, Yongey, 6, 74–80, 221–22
mirror neuron system, 144
mistakes, insight from, 156
money, as challenge to flourishing, 55–58
moral compass, 39
moral goodness, 39
moral retribution, 39
moral understanding and evaluation, 39
Morning Moments of Appreciation, 41
Mother Earth, relationship to, 220
motivation
    in challenging situations, 180
    for practice, 79, 91–92
    see also purpose
mundane moments
    Active Meditation–Finding Meaning in the Mundane, 254–55
    finding purpose in, 187–89, 194–95
    meaningful life vs., 179
    transformed into meaningful moments, 183
    see also daily life
Murthy, Vivek H., 52
Musk, Elon, 56

narratives constructed in the mind, *see* inner narratives
National Institutes of Health (NIH), 121–23
natural time cues, habits added to, 214–15
nature
    caring for, 178
    nurture vs., 61–63
    relationship to, 220
nature of reality, 84, 173
negative influences
    of inner narrative, 157
    knowing facts vs. myths about, 47
    news cycle as, 54–55
    obstacles to flourishing, 47 (*see also specific obstacles*)
Nepal, 175–79
nerve cells, 29–30
nervous system(s), 29–30
    of advanced meditators, 71
    social ties promoted by, 132
    threat response in, 151
neurodivergence, 67–68
neurons, 29, 32, 156
neuroplasticity, 25–32
    and brain changes, 26–29
    flourishing program's effect on, 60
    harnessing power of, 78

machinery of, 29–32
see also rewiring the brain
news cycle, 54–55, 118
New Yorker, The, 213
Nhat Hanh, Thich, 67
NIH (National Institutes of Health), 121–23
Noah, Trevor, 209–10
North Star, 180, 186
nurture, nature vs., 61–63
nurturing qualities, 141–42
    see also connection; *individual qualities*

objective connection, 126–27
object-oriented attention practices, 112–13
obstacles to flourishing, 47
    see also challenge(s)
Oishi, Shigehiro, 56–57
100th Birthday Party practice, 257
open awareness meditation, 79–80, 113–15
open-mindedness
    in defusing habitual responses, 159
    shifting from certainty to, 148 (*see also* insight)
open monitoring practice, 113
openness
    human preference for, 37
    to new possibilities, 84
    self-inquiry inviting, 159, 160
    see also curiosity
open presence meditation, 113
overwhelm
    causes of, 45–47
    forgetting habits of flourishing with, 226–27
    as outcome of evolutionary wiring, 45–46
    seeds of flourishing in, 24

pain
    advanced meditators' response to, 71
    brain's pain network, 15, 97–100, 142
    changing your experience of, 15, 221–22
    meditators' and non-meditators' responses to, 97–100
painting, awareness-based, 115
panic disorder, 76
parietal lobe, 67
Patan, Nepal, 175
path to flourishing, 67–94
    awareness in, 82
    connection in, 82–84
    and core dimensions of flourishing, 81–86

Index

path to flourishing (*cont.*)
  formal and informal practice in, 92–94
  framework for, 86–90
  insight in, 84–85
  and meditation research, 74–76
  mind training in, 79–81
  Mingyur Rinpoche in development of, 74–80
  people influencing development of, 68–74
  practices in, 76–79
  purpose in, 85–86
  transforming skills into practice in, 91–92
  see also Healthy Minds Framework; *specific skills*
perceived threats, 150–51
perception(s)
  curiosity challenging, 159
  examining, 153
  of income inequality, 57
  mind's influence on, 149
personal autonomy, as dimension of well-being, 184
personal growth, as dimension of well-being, 184
perspective-taking, self-inquiry linked to, 160
physical health
  connection for, 129
  eroded by worry and stress, 46
  flourishing skills' role in, 86
  and sense of purpose, 184, 200
  toll of chronic stress on, 151
physical movement, as gateway to awareness, 115
physiological needs, 56
planning
  self-inquiry linked to, 160
  Writing Reflection–Planning on Purpose, 256
pleasure, experience of, 69
pliability of brain and body, 25–26
poetry, awareness-based, 115
positive psychology, 84
positive relationships, as dimension of well-being, 184
post-traumatic growth, purpose and, 197–99
post-traumatic stress disorder (PTSD), 185, 197
power
  of awareness, 100–101
  of connection, 123–24
  of insight, 149–53
  of listening, 23

of neuroplasticity, 78
of purpose, 179–80
practice, in forming conscious habits, 213–14
practices for flourishing, 4, 12–15
  Active Meditation–Commuting with Connection, 245
  Active Meditation–Finding Meaning in the Mundane, 254–55
  Active Meditation–Morning Routine with Awareness, 239–40
  Active Meditation–Thoughts Shape Reality, 250
  awareness, 13, 17, 82, 103, 111–15, 235–42
  brain changes from, 27 (*see also* rewiring the brain)
  Compassionate Calendar, 140–41
  compassion practice, 14
  connection, 13, 82–84, 93, 129, 131–41, 235–36, 242–47
  in daily life, 15
  Distraction Reflection, 51
  epigenetic change from, 35–36
  formal and informal, 92–94
  growth through, 24
  Healthy Minds Index, 88–90
  Healthy Minds Meditation, 93–94, 235–36
  with Healthy Minds Program app, 17
  insight, 13, 17, 84–85, 235–36, 247–52
  Insight Through Dialogue, 168–69
  Interpersonal Practice–Exploring the Web of Causes and Conditions, 252
  Interpersonal Practice–Listening with Mindful Awareness, 241–42
  Interpersonal Practice–100th Birthday Party, 257
  Interpersonal Practice–Warm Memories, 247
  Journaling Reflection–Opportunities for Growth, 240–41
  Journaling to Nurture Kindness and Compassion, 139
  making time for, 226–27
  Morning Moments of Appreciation, 41
  Open Awareness Meditation, 113–15
  in path to flourishing, 76–79
  purpose, 13, 85–86, 182–83, 196–97, 235–36, 252–57
  for rewiring the brain, 41 (*see also* rewiring the brain)

simplicity and accessibility of, 14–15
Sitting Meditation–Breathing with
  Awareness, 237–39
Sitting Meditation–Extending Kindness
  in New Directions, 242–44
Sitting Meditation–Meaningful
  Memories, 252–54
Sitting Meditation–Opening to Change,
  247–49
Taste of Awareness, A, 103
Taste of Connection, A, 129
Taste of Insight, A, 154–55
Taste of Purpose, A, 182–83
time required for, 12–13, 219–20
transforming skills into, 91–92
Writing Reflection–Planning on
  Purpose, 256
Writing Reflection–Remembering
  Compassion, 246
Writing Reflection–What Leads to
  Growth and Insight?, 251
see also skills for flourishing; *specific practices*
prayer, awareness through, 115
prediction
  based on insight, 155–56
  as natural tendency, 156–57
prefrontal cortex, 53, 106, 226
presence, 8
  in awareness practices, 112
  in challenging situations, 100–101
  distraction vs., 50
  flourishing as, 16, 25
  with meta-awareness, 109
  mind's untapped potential for, 119
  open presence meditation, 113
  practicing, 105
  as quality of flourishing, 73
  skill of, 82 (*see also* awareness)
  in social interactions, 115–16
  Tibetan spiritual practices of, 74
  with wakeful awareness, 102–3
priorities
  recalibration of, 45
  in times of adversity, 186
procedural learning, 12
Proceedings of the National Academy of Sciences, 87
psychological well-being
  connection as core element of, 82
  and exposure to the news, 54
  sense of purpose for, 184

psychotherapy, as path to insight, 166–67
PTSD (post-traumatic stress disorder), 185, 197
"pure awareness," 80, 171
purpose, 8, 175–200
  action resulting from, 11
  in adversity, 184–87
  applied in daily life, 193–94
  in building a meaningful life, 199–200
  clarifying sense of, 180–82, 192–93
  cultivating, 92, 182–83
  in cultural analysis, 191
  defined, 11, 180
  as dimension of well-being, 184
  embodying your, 181, 193–94
  feeding your mind for, 190–92
  finding meaning in the mundane, 187–89
  five-minute daily practice for, 13
  flourishing as, 16, 25
  Healthy Minds Meditation for, 235–36
  human preference for, 37
  measuring, 88–90
  of Mingyur Rinpoche, 77
  in mundane and challenging situations, 194–95
  for older adults, 224–26
  in path to flourishing, 85–86
  and post-traumatic growth, 197–99
  power of, 179–80
  practices for, 13, 85–86, 182–83, 196–97, 235–36, 252–57
  pursuit of, 69
  as quality of flourishing, 73
  reflected in brain activity, 87
  research on, 11
  science of, 184
  as a skill, 192–95
  in theories of well-being, 86, 87
  through inner narrative, 157
  Tibetan spiritual practices of, 74
  in world's wisdom traditions, 81

questioning
  insight from, 161, 168–69
  in self-inquiry, 159

racism, brain's threat circuitry and, 54
reactions
  curiosity about, 151
  emotional (*see* emotional reactions/reactivity)
  insight into, 150, 151

reality
    Active Meditation–Thoughts Shape Reality, 250
    nature of, 84, 173
reflection
    daily rituals for, 191–92
    insight produced by, 85
    on typical flow of daily life, 212–13
reflective dialogue, as path to insight, 167
reflective writing
    as path to insight, 166
    reframing current challenge through, 196–97
    rewiring brain through, 13
    see also journaling; Writing Reflection
Reframe a Current Challenge, 196–97
relationship harmony
    art of, 82–84 (*see also* connection)
    and exposure to the news, 54
relaxation, human preference for, 37
reminders of skills, 226, 227
    see also cues
remote work, 52, 130–31
repetition, in developing habits, 213–14
research, 5–6
    on awareness practice, 31–32
    beyond mindfulness, 7
    on compassion practice, 14, 15
    on flourishing and well-being, 70 (*see also* path to flourishing)
    Healthy Minds Program app in, 18
    key insight from, 16
    on meditation, 74–76, 104
    on mindfulness, 87, 104
    at National Institutes of Health, 121–23
    on purpose, 184
    on rewiring the brain, 12–13
    on skills for flourishing, 8–11, 16 (*see also* individual skills)
    on smartphone addiction, 48
    on well-being, 86–87
    see also specific topics
resentment
    carrying, 136
    replacing, 145
resilience
    in challenging circumstances, 45
    flourishing as, 16
    helping others nurture, 222
    of mind, 191–92
    and mindfulness, 7
    and purpose, 11, 184, 187, 200
    research on, 7–8
    as response to challenges, 5
    rewiring brain for, 4
resting state brain activity, 117
reward network, 142
rewiring the brain, 21–41
    with awareness, 117–18
    and epigenetics, 32–36
    importance of intention in, 40
    and innate goodness, 36–40
    machinery of plasticity in, 29–32
    neuroplastic changes in, 26–29
    and pliability of brain and body, 25–26
    practice for, 4, 41
    through compassion practice, 14
    through meditation, 12–13, 71, 74–78
Ricard, Matthieu, 57
Rilke, Rainer Maria, 147
rituals, *see* daily rituals
Rosenkranz, Melissa, 35
routines
    Active Meditation–Morning Routine with Awareness, 239–40
    infused with intention, 204
    see also daily rituals; habits
Rumi
    on doing things from your soul, 175
    on helping others, 83
    on the present moment, 97
Ryff, Carol, 184

safety, need for, 56
salience network, 39, 106–8
security, need for, 56
self
    feeling compassion for, 138
    in flow experiences, 110–11
    sense/nature of, 84–85
self-acceptance, as dimension of well-being, 184
self-actualization, pursuit of, 69
self-awareness
    mindful, as decentering, 165
    self-knowledge vs., 164
self-compassion
    in observing inner narrative, 164
    practicing, 138
self-discovery
    building conscious habits for, 207
    insight as catalyst for, 149
    nurturing capacity for, 154
    in times of adversity, 187

Index

self-inquiry/exploration
    building conscious habits for, 207
    challenges as opportunities for, 23
    cultivating insight through, 84–85, 159–61
    in Healthy Minds Program, 174
    in Mahamudra, 70
    Tibetan spiritual practices of, 74
self-knowledge, 152
    combined with compassion and insight, 171
    nurturing capacity for, 154
    self-awareness vs., 164
    from self-inquiry, 159
self-mastery, awareness as ingredient of, 106, 111
self-reflection
    in clarifying purpose, 192–93
    in cultivating awareness, 115
    on failed relationships, 185
    self-inquiry as, 159 (*see also* self-inquiry/exploration)
    in times of adversity, 187
self-regulation
    brain regions responsible for, 117, 118
    cultivating conscious habits for, 206
    executive network in, 106
    salience network in, 107
    strengthened by connection, 144
    top-down, 106
self-transcendence, 152–53
self-transformation, in challenging situations, 180
sensory awareness, 116
sensory information integration, 67
sensory neurons, 29
serenity, in moments of deep flourishing, 24–25
Shamatha meditation, 173
Shantideva, 83
Shaw, George Bernard, 219
Sheinman, Nimrod, 223, 224
Singer, Tania, 160
Sitting Meditation
    Breathing with Awareness, 237–39
    Extending Kindness in New Directions, 242–44
    Meaningful Memories, 252–54
    Opening to Change, 247–49
skills for flourishing, 8, 10–11
    awareness, 82, 104–6
    brain changes with learning of, 31–32
    connection, 82–84, 130–31, 133–38
    innate capacity to develop, 9
    insight, 84–85, 161–63
    learning, 12 (*see also* practices for flourishing)
    making time to practice, 226–27
    measuring, 88–90
    purpose, 85–86, 192–97
    time required for, 219–20
    trainability of, 87
    transformed into practice, 91–92
    see also individual skills
sleep
    dreamless, 77
    gene expression and, 34
smartphones
    addiction to, 47–48
    as distraction, 48–50
smiling
    human preference for, 37
    as kindness, 125
social anxiety, loneliness and, 53
social comparison, 57–58
social connection, *see* connection
social interactions
    carrying resentment and frustration into, 136
    creating space for real connection in, 130–31
    elements of awareness in, 115–16
    feelings of connection in, 124–28, 130
    making time for skills practice around, 226–27
    negative and positive moments in, 131–32
    and well-being, 82
social isolation
    as challenge to flourishing, 52–53
    cultivating feelings of connection in, 127–28
social media, 5, 118
"soft skills," 142
South Africa, 210
stories, in the mind, *see* inner narratives
stress
    chronic, 45, 85, 151, 158
    compassion's effect on, 143
    current age of, 118–19
    early experiences of, 59
    and feeling of connection, 127
    moments of insight into, 151–52
    neuroscience of, 34

Index

stress (*cont.*)
    openness and curiosity in moments of, 160
    as outcome of evolutionary wiring, 45–46
    when distracted, 49
stressors, gene expression influenced by, 33, 34
stress reactions, 10
    and ability to grow new neurons, 32
    of advanced meditators, 71
stress reduction
    brain areas engaged in, 28
    five-minute daily practice for, 13
stress-related disorders, resilience as response to, 5
subjective connection, 126–27
subject-oriented attention practices, 113
suffering, 4
    beliefs leading to, 85
    experiencing pain without, 15, 99–100
    forgetting habits of flourishing when, 226–27
    forming healthy response to, 144
    relieving, 125 (*see also* compassion)
    self's relationship to, 85
    from stories created in the mind, 148, 149
    in training for compassion, 143
Sufi tradition, 115
suicide rates, 5, 18
support
    for connection, 126–29
    for flourishing, 45–46
    micro-, 215, 228
Swayambhu, Kathmandu, 175
systemic change, 220
systemic injustice, brain's threat circuitry and, 54

tai chi, 115
Taste of Awareness, A, 103
Taste of Connection, A, 129
Taste of Insight, A, 154–55
Taste of Purpose, A, 182–83
Tel Hai school, Israel, 223–24
Tergar International, 6, 259
Thoreau, Henry David, 115
thoughts
    about what is not happening, 50
    Active Meditation–Thoughts Shape Reality, 250
    of advanced meditators, 75
    awareness in managing, 106
    being present to your, 112
    curiosity and self-inquiry about, 159–60
    decentering in observation of, 164, 165
    in default-mode network, 158
    de-reification of, 164
    dysfunctional, 84
    harnessing power of, 158
    insight into, 8, 152
    positive, five-minute daily practice for, 13
    regulation of, 206
    sense of identity created with, 150
    that shape experience, 148
    toxic trains of, 107, 157, 158
    unhealthy, 85, 150
    see also inner narratives; mind
threat response, 151
threats
    brain circuitry detecting, 54–55
    perceived, 150–51
thriving
    building capacity for, 8
    sense of purpose for, 184
    by Tibetan monks, 72–73
    training ourselves for, 10
Tibet, 175
    refugees from, 175–78
    sense of purpose in culture of, 178
Tibetan Buddhism
    and propensity for goodness, 36–37
    "pure awareness" in, 171
    research on monks practicing, 70–73 (*see also* Mingyur Rinpoche, Yongey)
    teachers of, 6
top-down self-regulation, 106
toxic rumination, 157, 158
training, 9
    in awareness meditation, 31–32
    biology altered by, 61–62
    in compassion, 143–44
    of conscious habits, 205–6 (*see also* habits for flourishing)
    of the Dalai Lama, 124
    in emotion regulation, 160
    epigenetics altered by, 34–36
    to feel sense of direction in life, 85–86
    to flourish, 69–70, 79–81 (*see also* path to flourishing)
    with Healthy Minds Program app, 17
    interneuron growth and change from, 30
    of the mind, 27, 79–81
    in skills for flourishing, 87
    to widen connections, 83
    see also learning; practices for flourishing

Index

transcendent experiences, 152–53
trauma
    as challenge to flourishing, 58–60
    defined, 59
    gene expression influenced by, 33–34
    post-traumatic growth from, 197–99
    see also adversity
Tsoknyi Rinpoche, 221–22
twenty-four-hour news cycle, 54–55, 118
twin studies, 60

United States
    cultural trends in, 190–91
    declining life expectancy in, 46
    economic growth vs. well-being in, 55
    life expectancy in, 225
University College London, 30

values
    clarifying, 17
    communication of, 185
    conscious awareness of, 192
    in cultural analysis, 191
    of Mingyur Rinpoche, 76–77
    and sense of purpose in mundane situations, 187–89
virtues, in cultural analysis, 191
viscerotopic map, 28
vision
    for the awakening of all beings, 85
    for purpose in work, 182
visual cortex, 27–28
visualization, as cognitive maneuver, 67

warmth
    of the Dalai Lama, 123
    generating feelings of, 133, 134
    as quality of flourishing, 73
Way of a Pilgrim, The, 84
wealth, flourishing and, 55–58
well-being
    blind spots in research on, 86–87
    collective, crisis in, 18
    economic conditions and, 55

    emotional, 56–57, 125–26
    and feeling of support, 126–27
    hedonia vs. eudaimonia models of, 69
    heritability studies of, 61
    learning, 76
    meditation for, 5
    of Mingyur Rinpoche, 76
    most common challenge in cultivating, 204–5
    psychological, 54, 82, 184
    purpose as force for, 200
    rewiring brain for, 4
    sabotaged by inner narratives, 157
    scientific models of, 70, 104
    six dimensions of, 184
Weng, Helen, 143–44
Widom, Cathy, 59
willpower, awareness as ingredient of, 106
Wilson, Charlie, 213
wisdom, 5
    analytical meditations to cultivate, 80
    Dalai Lama on, 173
    from failed relationships, 185
    insight leading to, 84
    of Mingyur Rinpoche, 76
    as quality of flourishing, 73
    research on, 7–8
    of Tibetan monks, 72
    Tibetan spiritual practices of, 74
work
    knowing your purpose in, 180–82
    remote, 52, 130–31
world, problems facing, 118–19, 219–21
Wright, Erik Olin, 43–45
Writing Reflection
    Planning on Purpose, 256
    Remembering Compassion, 246
    What Leads to Growth and Insight?, 251
    see also reflective writing

Yehuda, Rachel, 33–34

zeitgebers, 214